11

WINNING

SECRETS

to STOP AGING

in its tracks

+ Bonus Material on The
Concierge Pt Method

By Dr. Sean T. Lordan, DPT

11 WINNING SECRETS TO STOP AGING IN ITS TRACKS

Copyright © 2021 By Dr. Sean T. Lordan, DPT

First paperback edition 2021

ACKNOWLEDGEMENTS

I would like to thank my wife Brooke, aunt Mary Lou, and mentor Bill DiBenedetto without whom none of this would be possible.

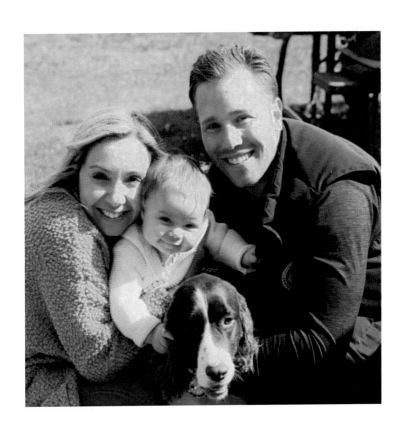

Dr. Sean T. Lordan, pictured with his wife, Brooke,
their daughter, Noelle, and their dog, Charlie

ABOUT THE AUTHOR

Dr. Sean T. Lordan PT, DPT, OCS, CSCS is a graduate of Northeastern University's Doctor of Physical Therapy (DPT) program. He is a specialist in Orthopedics certified by the American Physical Therapy Board of Physical Therapy Specialties (OCS). He is also recognized as a Certified Strength and Conditioning Specialist (CSCS) through the National Strength and Conditioning Association.

His clinical expertise ranges from treating pediatrics to geriatrics and includes Professional and Olympic athletes. He has made a habit of establishing routine protocols to help adjust and restore the body from the high demands of today's job market. He has practiced in California, Utah, and Georgia among other places in various clinical settings.

In 2016, Dr. Lordan started his own practice, Concierge Physical Therapy, treating patients in their homes in the Boston, MA area. He opened his first physical plant in 2018 in Sutton, MA where he was the sole Doctor of Physical Therapy.

Throughout his clinical endeavors, Dr. Lordan has treated a myriad of musculoskeletal disorders including repetitive trauma or overuse injury, tendonosis/itis, sciatica, low back pain, and patella-femoral dysfunction; all with successful outcomes. Another specialty in Dr. Lordan's repertoire is sport conditioning and rehabilitation, an area where he is able to specify personal treatment plans tailored to an individual's health and well-being. In this endeavor, he helps to reverse some of the deleterious effects of aging on the body's tissues.

The key to Dr. Lordan's concept is the Concierge Physical Therapy Regional Interdependence Model, which simply means that he approaches the body holistically. He treats patients with a total body perspective, not focusing on one joint at a time but rather the "bigger picture," to identify the root cause of a problem or injury.

TESTIMONIALS

I met Dr. Lordan when he started his PT Career in 2006, and joined the American Physical Therapy Association as just a Student PT...

From there he moved through Northeastern University's Accelerated Doctoral program and has spent the better part of the last 15 years perfecting a treatment approach different than conventional ones from the past...with proven success.

Working through the ranks from student to aide, to brand new PT to seasoned vet... all the way up to becoming a Board Certified Orthopedic Practitioner ....

And a member of the American Board of Physical Therapy Specialists...

He's now able to share the Concierge "Secret Success" formula with the world...

As well as Healthy Habits that will drastically reduce your risk for premature 'Aging'...

You may have seen him in the newspapers, on television, or on the internet doing podcasts and interviews... where he's frequently invited to share his opinion on current trends in the field of PT today... he is an invaluable resource to the PT community- and his patients don't realize how fortunate they are to have him.

-David Koehn, Owner, Boston Physical Therapy and Wellness

Sean and his staff at Concierge Physical Therapy are not only professional and friendly, but knowledgeable. Our experience has been over the top. My husband is on the road to recovery, and has avoided surgery. Sean was recommended to us, and so happy to be able to forward on to others our experience.

-Joy S., 64 y/o F

Highly professional staff! Very welcoming and family-like atmosphere. Dr. Sean and team got right to work on the physical therapy I needed. Perfect blend of consulting, therapy work, strengthening and coaching when I needed it most. I can't recommend them enough!

-Matt M., 50 y/o M

It took me 9 years to finally get myself to PT but my best decision was choosing Concierge! Everyone has been amazing and I look forward to every visit! I've only gone a few times but I can already feel a huge difference in my shoulder. I also love how they answer all my questions and explain everything in terms that I understand! Totally recommend to anyone!

-Demi M., 25 y/o F

BONUS ADDITIONS

At the time of writing, more than 50,000 people around the world receive regular and practical health information from me. My goal is to assist them in making sense of the very complicated world of 'tips' and 'healthy habits' provided by gurus from every continent. Let me help YOU. Subscribe today and claim your tips which includes lots of information targeted to those over the age of 50.

It is easy to do. Just go to conciergephysicaltherapy.com and download one or more free reports: Knee/ Shoulder/ Low Back/ Anti-Aging... whichever ones are of interest to you. If you choose the 'Gifts' pathway, fill out the form on the screen and I will send you some goodies and gifts. All for signing up! The gifts include a myriad of health information and a 7- step guide to Anti-Aging and building a healthier and happier 'you.' This is perfect for ANY person aged 50 or older who is looking to remain pliable into the golden years. You will be able to access them right away when you enter your name and email to www.conciergephysical-therapy.com/gifts.

If you follow the simple instructions in my guides, you WILL notice a difference in how healthy you look and feel. Go to www.conciergephysicaltherapy.com/gifts to make sure you receive them. There will be more gifts to follow over the coming months and years. Don't miss out. Enroll and be on the email list!

FOREWARD

This entire book hinges upon one key belief that I have settled on after years of practice and know to be the only solution to the problems ailing our baby boomer generation and beyond.

A holistic total-body approach is the key to keeping your body healthy and active well into old age. It is attainable through a Regional Interdependence Model, much like the one we use at Concierge Physical Therapy.

What is the concept of 'Regional Interdependence' you ask? I will cover that concept in more detail throughout the chapters of this book. For now, simply put, regional interdependence refers to how all of the systems of your body work together in concert to produce movement, thoughts and your current level of well-being and consciousness.

I will delve into the total body approach technique throughout the course of this book. The solution you have been looking for when it comes to living the life that you've always dreamed of is not out of reach. Quite the contrary, it is now ever closer to your grasp. This book covers topics including nutrition, exercise, mental health and wellness while offering practical tips in language and anecdotes that are easy to understand. Also included are certain tips from my years of clinical expertise to help you or a loved one eradicate back, shoulder and knee pain.

CONTENTS

MASTER THE MINDSET

By design, my book is a manual providing clarity for those who are aged fifty plus who are looking to live a more active and healthier lifestyle. It is also meant to enlighten the reader with the goal of preventing the use of walkers, canes and wheelchairs down the line. The reader is strongly encouraged to accept the theory of a growth mindset.

Having this type of mindset is a key marker to success in many chapters of our lives. It is also a key component in challenging the status quo of medical advice offered today. The advice in my book is written for those who refuse to give in to the assumption that the second half of life is a time of progressive deterioration. Your retirement years should be a time of great opportunity. Your golden years should be enjoyed by enhancing your lifestyle, mental state and overall well-being. Please keep an open mind while reading and implementing the healthy habits outlined in my book. If you read closely you may find at least one tip that could change your life.

My advice is to start small and implement two to three of the suggestions offered. If you can successfully accomplish that you will be well on your way to a happier and healthier life - a life with joyous fulfillment and many blessed days to come!

Due to advancements in science and technology we, especially in America, have the ability to live into our eighties, nineties and beyond. We can also now live with a better quality of life than was ever thought possible. Those who do so employ a little bit of self-discipline and a few of the 'winning rules' from this book.

Mobility, strength and mental acuity are all part of the human experience and critical aspects of our health. Each one is adaptable and with practice can be improved upon. Concentrating on these areas will lead to a more independent and fulfilling lifestyle well into old age.

In order to improve mobility, strength and mental acuity a certain level of self-discipline is required. Self-discipline indicates a structured, well thought out and consistent approach to your health. According to an old saying, "practice makes perfect." Unfortunately, many people are missing out on easy opportunities to improve their quality of life and overall health. The obvious question is: Why?

This book intends to answer some health questions that are of greatest concern to you by walking you through some easy tips. Tips that are essential to having a long, healthy life free of medications, pills and unnecessary surgeries that plague many of your friends and loved ones. Again by design, it is also a guide to help make your lifestyle choices easier if you are looking for this outcome: *a healthier overall life experience today and in the future.*

3 Saboteurs of a Healthy Lifestyle

Let's talk about a few of the saboteurs that can get in your way preventing you from living your "best life." I will touch on a few in the introduction and delve a little bit deeper the further we go in this book. From my experience, I find there are **(3)** main reasons your health could be compromised.

1. **The 'It Must Be My Age' Mindset.** At the first sign of pain, stiffness or muscle ache many people just accept it as reality and think, "This must be my age; I'm just getting old." Many will self-medicate to make the symptoms go away without ever addressing the root cause. It is essential to determine if it is a core strength issue, or is there something underlying or concomitant going on? What complicates matters further is that some of the exercises or activities that relieve your pain and symptomatology will hurt a little bit! You need a good coach to help get you through the grind. It also helps to have a medical professional clearly explain why you should push through a pain threshold. For example, there is a positive correlation between performing specific exercises and a reduction in joint pain caused by arthritis.

2. **Poor Advice and Self-Diagnosis:** Not everything you read on the internet is true. Bad advice may be a leading intruder that is sabotaging your personal health journey. With access to a wealth of information (WebMD, Wikipedia) many people are turning to the quick and easy way, but not the right way, to solve a healthcare problem. They tend to self-diagnose. People often are doing so prior to consultation with a Primary Care Physician (PCP) or specialist. Just because you may have a professional degree in another field does not mean that you

have the years of experience a Primary Care Healthcare Practitioner has obtained. You wouldn't ask your accountant for legal advice. Why would you ask google how to fix your back pain?

Please take a moment to consider how dangerous self-diagnosing can be. What if you miss obvious signs of cancer or a neurological disease because WebMD tells you that your symptoms are normal? Conversely, what if the shooting pain down your legs is not "Sciatica" but a malignant tumor on your L5 nerve root that can only be properly diagnosed with an X-Ray and /or MRI? Unfortunately, there is often confirmation bias involved in self-diagnostics. Confirmation bias occurs when you *think* you have sciatica, google the results, and convince yourself that you have other side effects as well, supposedly confirming your self-diagnosis. There is a reason the most trusted Healthcare Providers obtain Doctorate Degrees!

Those who are searching online for quick solutions pay a much higher price in the long term. Following years of education and research, medical practitioners often find it challenging to determine what is wrong. How can a non-healthcare provider think that they can do better? A study by Graber et. al. in 2012 indicates that diagnostic errors can be present up to 20% of the time at the PCP level! Let me ask you to consider the following: "If your doctor can only get the diagnosis right 80% of the time, do you think you will obtain more accurate information on WebMD?" (If so please email me your lottery picks as well because you must be very lucky!) My point is: the quick, cheap and easy solution often leads to a longer more costly result. This is particularly true when it comes to commercial healthcare and rising deductibles.

3. **Need for Instant Gratification.** Instant gratification is killing Baby Boomers, Millennials, and Gen X'ers. More often than not, people are putting off long term goals for short term ephemeral happiness. Let's consider Amazon for instance. We can now have packages delivered the same day for free. Why bother with the inconvenience of going to the store when we can sit at the computer and just click a button?

In medicine, the need for instant gratification is also ingrained in our psyche. Do you have a headache? Take an aspirin and ten minutes later your headache is gone. However, the topic of weight loss is a whole different proverbial ball-game. When I tell a patient it takes 3-6 months to truly make a change, I have instantly lost my audience. When directed to "lose weight" by their Primary Care Physicians many are left unsure about what steps to actually take to make weight loss come to fruition. Couple that with physicians' bias of negative attitudes and beliefs concerning their overweight or obese patient's ability to adhere to medical recommendations (Pool et al. 2003), and we have a medical conundrum.

The science overwhelmingly points to a direct relationship of obesity to the incidence of low back and knee pain. Although most people are aware that carrying excess abdominal adiposity puts more pressure on their joints and organs, few are willing to take the long term steps to actually do something about it. Why not just put on a pain patch, or rub some CBD oil in, or take a pain pill. The thought process is: This will provide immediate relief and get me back to normal. Unfortunately, the more you ignore a health problem, and more importantly, its root cause, the harder it is to fix. Do you see where I am headed with this?

Losing weight takes time and requires a significant amount of self-discipline and will-power. Most people are simply unable to visualize themselves in one year's time in a slimmer pair of pants or slacks living a healthier and more fulfilling lifestyle. All it takes is one step in the right direction to help solve that problem today.

If a person with chronic pain and activity-limiting arthritis is unable to resist pleasurable experiences, such as eating chocolate bars, brownies and muffins, they must identify the problem as a first step. When folks continue to make poor decisions causing more pain and suffering, the proper choices will become readily apparent. The decision then becomes the right choice versus the wrong choice. What chance do they have of living a healthy life into their eighties, nineties and beyond if they continue to knowingly make the wrong choices when it comes to their nutrition and health? The question is: How do you qualify the scope of your nutrition problem and the poor decisions you are making? How do your mealtime choices affect your overall longevity? This book will help identify ways to self reflect and ultimately change your poor habits to achieve the desired outcome of aging gracefully, with full independence, mobility and strength not only intact but thriving!

Smart Choices versus Easy Choices

My book is packed with unique health secrets; the type you will not learn in your PCP's office or on WebMD. Your ability to maintain independence, strength and mobility into your senior years, free from painkillers and surgery hinges upon your ability to make smart choices. Smart choices are not always easy choices. Making a smart choice and overcoming your own self-destructive tendencies are the keys to creating the positive change in your lifestyle that you are seeking. It is only through a model of self-discipline that you will be able to make positive changes in your life. Self-discipline hinges on consciously avoiding the easy choice, and instead making the smart choice that you intuitively know is the right one. Self-discipline is the plan. Will-power is the action. It takes a plan of self-discipline to say to yourself: "I'm going to live a healthier life." It takes will-power to choose a protein shake instead of a donut for breakfast. It takes will-power to decide to walk around the neighborhood during a conference call instead of taking the call while sitting at your desk.

Your health decisions will be infinitely easier if you have reliable information from a specialist at your fingertips. My job is to help to make your new habits and decisions simple and easy to follow. That is the essence of this book.

What Should you Expect from Reading this Book?

If you follow the practical tips laid out in my book, you will see a rise in your life expectancy and an improvement in the quality of your life. *It's that simple.*

You will feel better, move more fluidly and be a better version of yourself than you currently are today. Even if you 'like' yourself today, by implementing some of these tips, you will 'love' yourself in a short period of time. Simply implement a few of the tips that are located on these pages and you will experience a significant lifestyle change for the better. What is stopping you now from becoming the best version of *you?* Only yourself!

CHAPTER ONE

MAKE THE RIGHT CHOICE WITH YOUR HEALTH

It is important to note that living a healthy lifestyle is about making the right decision at the right time. Relying on the latest pharmaceuticals to become a cure for a future illness, you may or may not acquire, is not a plausible solution. Using the tools I outline will enable you to make the right choices when it comes to your health. You will be able to understand the immediate and long term consequences of each decision you make. The good news is that you are off to a good start by reading my book!

Let's start with a simple 'decision making' example:

I'd like to introduce Jan, a 65 year old woman who recently retired and is twenty pounds overweight. She suffers from chronic hip, knee and low back pain. While her hobbies include gardening and skiing, she hasn't been able to do either in recent years due to increasing pain. Her knees click when she walks up and down stairs and her back aches after walking only a short distance, a quarter mile or so. She is no longer able to engage in the activities she enjoys. But, because she has no "chronic" conditions like diabetes or COPD, she considers herself better off than many of her contemporaries. She has never had a full body physical assessment from a Physical Therapist to discuss her inability to continue enjoying the activities that bring her happiness. However, she does pride herself upon going to her Primary Care Physician at least once a year for standard testing and a review of blood work. Jan knows that she needs to do something about her nagging aches and pains, but is unsure where to start. I suggest that Jan would benefit greatly from just a few simple habit exchanges in her daily life. These habits will help to improve her quality of life and overall happiness.

Jan's 'Get Healthy' Program in 3 steps

Jan's first step to becoming healthy would encompass a walking program beginning with a loop around the neighborhood everyday for 20-30 minutes. This will help improve her blood circulation bringing critical elements like oxygen and endorphins to the brain and muscles that cause the post workout euphoria that many of us experience.

Jan's second step should be to schedule a one-hour consultation with a Physical Therapist who will help Jan to see where her body needs stretching and strengthening. During the first session Jan will learn 3-4 simple exercises to incorporate into her daily routine to improve strength in the areas of her body where she experiences weakness and tightness. In order to eliminate aches or pains, it is essential to identify the *cause* of the symptoms. The root cause of Jan's symptoms likely may not be in the same area of her body that is presenting with pain and dysfunction. For that reason, it is critical for Jan to get a proper full body assessment to make sure she is doing all she can to prevent premature arthritic decay of joints and surfaces of her body.

The third step Jan could take is to begin tracking her daily caloric intake. There are many ways to do this now with a plethora of applications that focus on this alone. My favorite apps are *Noom, cronometer* and *myfitnesspal.* In order to achieve maximum results from this exercise, I would recommend that Jan track all of the food she eats for three days. Doing so will allow her to see what she is actually consuming and encourage her to reflect on whether it is sabotaging her goals of losing weight and staying physically fit.

Three simple steps, all requiring self-discipline and will-power. Pursuing this strategy will allow Jan to drop the excess weight that is contributing to her aches and pains. She will lose abdominal fat (which is linked to an increase in risk for many cancers according the *US News and World Report*), and subsequently she will report higher levels of life satisfaction. What does life satisfaction translate to for Jan? Sociability with her friends, gardening and skiing are among her favorites. Jan will be able to do what she loves for longer periods of time if she begins with those three steps! What does your three step program look like? Well, let's see if I can assist you in making that determination.

Compounding Healthy Habits with Will Power and Inertia

In order to compound Healthy Habits, it is easiest to take one negative decision and replace it with a positive one. The goal is to start small so that the process does not become overwhelming. For example: you may choose to go to the gym for an hour and participate in a strength class instead of binge watching *Queen's Gambit* on Netflix. One positive decision swapped for a negative decision.

We all perform our daily tasks with a certain level of inertia and mindlessness. Think about brushing your teeth in the morning. Do you wake up and think, "should I brush my teeth today?" or, do you just perform the act of brushing without thinking about it as part of the inertia that started when you rolled out of bed?

Inertia is what helps us stack habits whether they be positive or negative. Will-power is what helps us create and sustain a positive habit. If you are used to sitting on the couch after work everyday (daily inertia), the initial decision to go to the gym (requiring will-power) will be the most difficult one. The first decision in the series will be the most difficult because it requires strong will-power.

Will-power has the tendency to diminish over the course of the day. You were tempted by the donuts at work in the morning, but you persevered and didn't have one. With only a certain amount available each day, your will-power has now diminished! Next, you had a Kale salad with apples and balsamic vinaigrette for lunch even though the store had a very tempting display of Italian subs that you were salivating over. Your daily amount of will-power is now further diminished. The remaining will-power will probably not be sufficient to motivate you to spend 30 minutes on the Peloton when you get home from work! After all, you were able to say no to the doughnuts and Italian subs. Haven't you earned the right to binge watch TV while enjoying a bowl of Ben and Jerry's?

NO! But we believe we are because this is sadly how we are 'wired!'

Healthy Habit Winning Rule #1: You must first use will-power to make a positive decision affecting your health. Then inertia will help make this positive change *permanent*.

How to Improve Will Power

What affects your ability to improve your will-power? What do those with a lot of will-power have in common? Those that have strong will-power are able to accurately self-reflect on what they want most out of life. They are also able to demonstrate delayed gratification at a higher rate than others. Providing evidence of this theory is a famous experiment performed in the 1960's dubbed the "Marshmallow Experiment."

The Marshmallow experiment was performed by esteemed psychologist Walter Mischel. He offered 4-year-olds the choice of one marshmallow now, or two if they could wait 15 minutes. He and other researchers then tracked the performance of these children as they became adults. They found that children who resisted temptation ("high delayers") achieved greater academic success (higher SAT scores), better health (lower BMI), and lower rates of marital separation and divorce. Mischel concluded that the ability to delay gratification constituted "*a protective buffer against the development of all kinds of vulnerabilities later in life.*"

The ability to delay gratification is only one marker identified in the development of a rock solid will-power. To delve further, it is important to understand how will-power works. Will-power works in a manner similar to the muscles in your body. Just as a muscle becomes exhausted after a workout, your will-power, too, may become 'exhausted.' But, will-power will strengthen in resolve when used in the appropriate frequency and duration. In order to reserve stamina, you wouldn't lift weights for two hours in your home gym prior to running a marathon. Similarly, our will-power has a stamina component too.

In order to maximize the effects of will-power we should begin to change our habits in small increments. I suggest beginning a new 15 minute daily exercise circuit to start training your will-power. This is not a large time commitment and can easily be worked into a morning, mid-day or nighttime routine for even the busiest folks. You should aim to try this for three weeks.

Once the first habit is in place, the 15-minute exercise routine, no *excess* will-power is required to perform it. You are building inertia! The exercise routine has become a new healthy habit. Now let's leverage the power of inertia and habit stacking.

Inertia and Habit Stacking

Habit stacking is a powerful strategy to help merge activities in order to magnify the outcome, often from just a small investment of will-power. Considering it took a substantial amount of will-power for a few weeks to develop your new exercise habit, you have now successfully recovered your reservoir and are able to use your will-power reserve again. Since you are feeling so well from working out, you choose to eat a grilled chicken salad accompanied by a large glass of ice water immediately afterward. Although you would much rather a cheeseburger and fries, you decide that it is best for your well being (use of will-power) to have the grilled chicken salad. Continue this trial for a few days and see if it will stick. My experience indicates that it does! Just like that you have stacked two positive habits. You have learned to use the inertia from a quick workout routine and the benefits of habit stacking from reading this book. You are well on your way to success! Sounds too easy to be true... right?

Dangers of Inertia and Will Power Depletion

Lacking a strong will-power, inertia is a dangerous force that will perpetuate bad habits. That is why it's crucial to do what we can to train our will-power to allow us to make better choices from day to day. We naturally tend to look for the path of least resistance, at work and at home. In the world of Physical Therapy, we often see injuries that occur in the direction of the "path of least resistance" because this is where a joint capsule is most exposed. Many find it much easier to prop-up their heels in a recliner than to ride a Peloton bike for 30 minutes. That is the danger of inertia. Having a bad day? Have a *Snickers*. That will make you feel better, right? Unfortunately, no. Science supports the idea that carbohydrates actually give us the same mental affects (stimulate the same neurotransmitters) as opiate analgesics. Does that sound crazy? Carbohydrates can be just as addictive as opiates. It all depends on how we condition our brain's reward systems to cope with our lifestyle.

Is your Brain a Friend or a Foe?

The quick answer is: It depends! In order to maintain proper brain chemistry and reward pathways, it is crucial to stay committed on a daily basis to positive habits. Your brain and body get used to the current way you do things (homeostasis). Your brain is wired to reward any activity it gets pleasure from, and it does so using the neurotransmitters dopamine and serotonin. There are many other neurotransmitters involved in reshaping your habits, but I will keep it to the main two for the sake of brevity. The art of your brain's role in changing your habits is called neuroplasticity. Neuroplasticity refers to the way your brain changes over time to adapt to stimulus from the outside world.

During and after an intense workout, the rush of endorphins you feel is also accompanied by a cascade of dopamine, serotonin and norepinephrine in your brain. The endorphins help relieve pain and stress and the other neurotransmitters help to give you a sense of accomplishment after completing your workout. Regular exercise also helps to regulate the release of serotonin which is an important neurotransmitter involved in mood stabilization and increasing your sense of well-being.

Some ways to improve your body's regulation and modulation of serotonin and dopamine in order to feel an immediate positive affect on your mood include:

1. Exercising Daily
2. Going for a Walk in Nature

3. Eating a Well-Balanced Nutritious Diet
4. Meditating Daily
5. Practicing Daily Gratitude

Let's talk about your brain's ability to create a negative habit. Think about any addiction. For instance, when a drug addict uses heroin, it stimulates an immediate cascade of endorphin release in the brain. This release is one which the brain begins to crave more as the user continues perpetual use. This is referred to as neurological adaptation. Eventually the drug addict uses more and more of the narcotic to satisfy the brain's receptors, but the endorphin rush feels about the same or is diminished each time. This is a prime example of how your brain becomes reliant on a negative habit and can truly become a "foe."

The same can be said about a similar negative feedback loop, eating fast food. Eating a *McDonald's* quarter pounder will immediately satisfy your desire for salt and fat, two nutrients we are wired from a young age to value above others. When your body receives these nutrients, it craves more. You continue the habit to create the ephemeral rush of endorphins. This rush however doesn't last long because about an hour later, if your are similar to me, you feel a bit sick to your stomach. You will notice the longer you go without fast food, the worse you feel after reintroducing it to your diet. The reason is your body and brain are not conditioned to eating salt, fat and preservatives in such quantities, and a stomach ache is your body's way of rejecting it.

Here are some tips to get the most out of this book. Please have a pen and paper or a highlighter ready to use. I will highlight the tips in bold so that they are easy to remember and refer to.

Tip One: Keep an open mind. Throughout the book you will read things that will not make sense to you, or that are not in line with what you may have learned in the past from mainstream medicine. What I'm asking is that you give these tips a chance. Just *try them out.* Some advice may work for you, some may not, but at least give it a shot.

Tip Two: Try something new. In line with the first tip, please do not be afraid to try something new. This can be as simple as going on a hike for the first time, or perhaps going for your first swim. The advice in my book is meant to take you out of your comfort zone and into an area that will push you to be a healthier version of yourself. Do yourself a favor and TRY it! If you don't like it that is okay, but I challenge you to implement at least one or two Healthy Habits in your life. Then see the dramatic changes that unfold over time.

Tip Three: Implement at least ONE habit from this book. My challenge to you is to implement just ONE habit from this book and stay with it for 21 days. If you can do that then you are much more likely, from a psychological perspective, to stack good habits on top of the ONE that you chose. You will be setting yourself up for success in the future!

> The key is consistency... and small targeted habits that, when executed consistently, add up to profound results.

CHAPTER TWO

THE PATH TO A LIFE WELL LIVED: AVOIDING COMMON PITFALLS

When my patient, Jim, first came to my clinic, he commented: "Dr. Lordan, I often find myself going from one exercise fad to another- but nothing ever seems to 'stick'. I get bored easily and sometimes I just totally forget to do some of the simple things I even enjoy- like going on a nightly stroll around my neighborhood with my wife. Worse, when I take weeks off at a time, I find it even harder to start up a routine again. I experience stiffness and aches afterwards. So I have two questions: Is it normal to get 'stiff' after not exercising for a while? And how do I find the motivation to keep active on a daily basis?"

Here is the advice I gave Jim: Find the reason WHY you're exercising in the first place. The first question you will have to answer in order to find the intrinsic motivation to keep going, along with the drive to exercise is: What is it that you are looking to gain from exercise? Or, maybe there is an outcome you are trying to avoid by exercising. Perhaps you have an aging family member in the hospital who isn't doing well, or ones who have lost all of their independence and rely on other people to assist with tasks such as meal preparation, personal hygiene, or going to the bathroom. You do not want to end up like them! Fear is a powerful motivator. It is NORMAL to be afraid of having a joint replacement or spinal surgery! To tie it all back to your question, Jim, in order to find the motivation to exercise, you need to think of what it is you truly want to gain from being more active. It is OK if your answer is to simply be able to 'move with less stiffness' or to reduce your risk for disease. However, these outcomes are less tangible and may not give you the inertia to move you during crunch time.

Conversely, let's put into perspective what life would look like if you don't exercise. We know that exercise has a host of benefits including, but not limited to: improved weight loss (by increasing metabolism), improved mood (through endorphins), increased strength, improved vascularity and blood flow, and improved mental acuity. That is only the start. If you do not exercise, we know that you will not get any of the benefits listed above. Then you will be facing the consequences of being a couch potato.

Research shows the effects of not exercising and living a sedentary lifestyle are daunting. Those who do not exercise are often classified at a higher risk for mortality due to the common conditions associated with that type of lifestyle.

These conditions include: high blood pressure, diabetes, cardiovascular disease, greater risk for heart attack and stroke, depression, insomnia, obesity, osteoporosis (poor bone density) and idiopathic scoliosis.

20

The questions you should be asking yourself, Jim, are: Is it worth it? Is it worth the potential downside of becoming obese, depressed and at a higher risk for a heart attack or stroke? Or is it worth the effort to go to the gym or for a walk three nights a week? When I put it that way, does it provide some motivation to work out, Jim? Hopefully you have some fuel and incentive for when it is 10 degrees outside in the dead of winter. You really NEED to go for a walk or get to the gym keeping in mind what could happen if you do not!

Lessons Learned from your Aged Loved One

When people in their 40s, 50s and 60s come to see me at my outpatient PT clinic, they often reference their parents or ailing loved ones. They do not want to follow the same path that genetics seemingly laid out for their predecessors. I get the impression they worry that it will not be too long before the effects of not exercising impact them as well. Obviously that is not what anyone wants. Often people start to realize this while in my PT clinic. During the initial PT 'Evaluation' when consulting with a Doctor of Physical Therapy, many people START to acknowledge what they need to do to avoid becoming inactive or immobile.

As a practitioner it is disheartening and often frustrating to see what 'could have been' for an aging adult if only they had lived a healthier lifestyle. I am fairly confident that even folks who do not talk about losing independence must think about it on occasion. Do you? It's human nature to worry. Luckily, with the advent of the internet and 5G services we have a myriad of health information at our fingertips putting us in a much better position to make healthier decisions with the assistance of a PCP or PT than our parents' generation had.

Make the Most Out of Life

I have a client in his 90's named Ron who comes to see me regularly at Concierge. He is from Sutton, MA where one of my PT Clinics is located. I want you to know a little bit about him so you can perhaps emulate his habits and way of thinking. Having no immediate family, Ron must maintain his mobility and independence by himself. His only aid is an electric scooter. His social support structure is small, so he cannot rely on others for the daily necessities (grocery shopping/ trips to the laundromat, etc.) that many of us take for granted. When Ron wants to go for a swim, he walks to the bus stop and waits for transportation to the YMCA. Swimming is an excellent habit because it is easy on the bones and joints while giving the cardiovascular and pulmonary systems an excellent workout. Without exercise, those systems can be the first to fail in old age. The social interaction Ron enjoys with the friends he has made is an added bonus he receives every time he goes to the YMCA to swim. The benefits of social interaction for Ron cannot be understated. They keep his mind sharp and his attitude positive. I marvel at his ability to converse about anything from current events to politics. His mind is keen and open to new perspectives and angles. Social interaction is key to positive neuroplastic changes that allow his brain to stay healthy while warding off dementia and cognitive decay.

Most would agree that there is a certain level of 'luck' involved in reaching the age of 92. However, I believe Ron helped 'create luck' with positive daily habits performed over a considerable amount of time. Ron began swimming at age 60, so he has been swimming now for 30+ years! Ron's self proclaimed health secret is: "I simply exercised at the same time everyday- it was never

hard- I never had to 'make a decision.' I just went out and did it."
So I urge you to take a page out of Ron's book. Stick with one
positive habit and do it at the same time everyday. The cumulative
effects will astound you.

Fall Prevention Techniques, a Strategy and a Mindset

Next, I'd like to share some easy tips and advice for you to start
on right away while you are reading this book. These tips will help
you protect and strengthen your joints and muscles. They will
help you remain fit and active while improving your ability to
exercise in a way you never have before.

Let's tackle a common complaint affecting those who are 60+,
especially those living through the harsh New England winters:
fear of falling. The statistics related to falls are mind-boggling.
According to the *World Health Organization,* an estimated
646,000 individuals around the globe die yearly from falls. Adults
older than 65 years of age suffer the greatest number of
fatal falls. Thirty-seven point three (37.3) million falls that are
severe enough to require medical attention occur each year.
With so many simple prevention strategies, it is staggering that
falls are such an epidemic, especially in the United States. Among
the most common preventable causes of falls include: an unsafe
environment (throw rugs, loose cords etc. in the home), poor
mobility, lack of a consistent strength program, unsafe use of
assistive devices (canes/ walkers) and lack of follow up with a
Pharmacist and Primary Care regarding poly-pharmacy (taking
too many meds). YES, it is normal to be afraid of falling and to
feel 'unsteady' on your feet. Let's delve into what I see in the clinic
and what you can do to prevent yourself from becoming a WHO
statistic.

A common patient complaint, that I look at as an opportunity to be of help, is feeling unsteady on your feet as you age. This can be caused by one or more factors, such as: a lack of balance stemming from a breakdown in your vision, your vestibular system (more on this later), or the sensation at the bottom of your feet. The good news is that all of these bodily systems are adaptable and can change based on your willingness to train them. I have included some simple balance exercises in the appendix of this book. Try them if this is a condition that applies to you.

As a Healthcare provider, how do I treat balance issues? One of the **first things** that I look at is the type of footwear a patient is wearing. This simple observation has helped me to improve countless lives by offering advice about the necessity of wearing appropriate shoes. For some, I recommend the addition of inserts which can improve gait and balance significantly.

What NOT to Wear On Your Feet

When it comes to a healthy exercise routine, walking is one of the best conditioning programs around. I recommend walking on varied surfaces at varied inclines to get the most 'bang for your buck' when it comes to cardiovascular benefits. When your body encounters a new training surface (grass, mulch, dirt, tarmac) it subconsciously has to adapt to that surface using a unique muscle combination, known as your sensory-motor system, each time. Your feet use a technique called "pronation" to adapt to each type of surface you walk on which helps to absorb shock and reduce the 'pounding effect' that walking has on your joints. Pronation is a normal phenomenon. Without it your body would ache due to a stiff ankle and foot joint delivering shocks 'up the chain' and prove to be extremely taxing on your knees, hips and back!

If 'looking good' is your main priority in shoe selection, chances are that your HSA or FSA account will be drained by the time you reach retirement. Fancy high heels and flats often lead to a variety of problems for your feet by propagating the bunion effect and throwing off joint mechanics all the way up to the spine. This is simply because of a lack of 'cushioning' which places the foot in a position to absorb more shock as a rigid lever. I believe most people know that shoes providing a 'cushion' are generally better for your feet than flat shoes or rigid ones. There are some exceptions. What often goes unnoticed is how shoes are worn. Are they loose leaving your joints able to rub up against surfaces and spots that they shouldn't? Are you tying the laces too tight potentially cutting off circulation to pivotal spots in the foot? These details definitely matter when it comes to footwear and the selection of the appropriate shoes to wear on a daily basis. Most people do not know that they could prevent a bunion from getting worse simply by buying a more supportive shoe or using orthotic insoles.

My point is, unless you have seen a Podiatrist, Chiropractor or Physical Therapist lately, the chances that footwear is on your list of 'Healthy Habits' to change is slim to none. Most folks are unaware of the benefits a simple upgrade in footwear can have on your overall health. Statistics show that 70% of Americans have flat feet. Most cases of flat feet contribute to pain in the knees, hips and low back. If just a fraction of those people read this book and look into orthotic inserts or more supportive footwear, they will reduce their risk of joint disease later in life! I strongly suggest consulting your local Physical Therapist prior to changing your footwear. They will do a gait analysis, tell you whether or not a change is needed, and make suggestions about appropriate selections.

CHAPTER THREE

HOW TO FIND 7 DAYS WORTH OF SPARE TIME

According to a recent study reported in the *NY Post* the average person spends 36 years of life in bed! This staggering statistic was arrived at by adding up the number of hours we typically sleep (about 7 hours) to the time we sit in bed watching Netflix and other shows (around 4 hours). For many that equates to 11 hours of lounging a day. 11 hours! What an incredible opportunity this is to find time in your day to spend productively. What could you accomplish with 4 more hours a day? Wouldn't it be nice to have an extra 20 hours during the Monday through Friday work week? I'm not suggesting that you sleep less than 7 hours a night. But think about the opportunity those 4 hours of sitting in bed provide. Interestingly, it has been widely reported that sleeping more than 7 hours a night might even be deleterious to your health! So who knows what to believe? Do you need 8-10 hours of sleep per night, or is 7 actually better? The answer is, it depends on the sleep habits you create and what your body becomes used to.

This "Netflix and Chill" phenomena gets worse in the winter months when the days are shorter and it is much more difficult to leave your cozy bedroom to deal with the subzero temperatures looming outside your front door. The best way to manage a sleep strategy is to go to sleep at the same time every night and wake up at the same time every morning. If you are able to do so consistently (while getting 7 hours minimum) you will feel less lethargic and have more energy when you wake up. I highly recommend that you Do NOT, I repeat: Do NOT! touch the snooze button on your alarm clock. Doing so is the number one waste of time in the morning. On top of the poor quality of sleep you receive during this time, you are wasting precious minutes that you could spend having a leisurely breakfast or enjoying quality family time.

If you are currently sleeping 10 hours a night, try to gradually reduce the number to 7 or 8 hours (which is all your body most likely needs). If you combine the 2 hours you gain from sleeping less, with the 4 hours you can potentially gain from eliminating the habit of lying in bed watching television, that's a whopping 6 extra hours a day! At that rate you can find **extra time amounting to a week in just one month**!

> **Healthy Habit Winning Rule #2:** Get out of bed ONE hour earlier each morning and spend it doing something you ENJOY.

5 Tips to Wake Up Like a Rockstar

Are you winning or losing the "battle of the bedroom?" Do you wake up in the morning feeling groggy and agitated? Is your sleep interrupted by a partners snoring, or dogs barking (or cats meowing)? Here are a few simple tips to help you wake up refreshed and improve your daily outlook.

1.) If you're going to bed at 10pm or later, **aim to stop eating after 5pm.** If you absolutely have to eat, have a protein shake or something easily digested. This will diminish the chance that your digestive system will keep you awake as it works to digest a heavy lasagna meal or steak dish.

2.) **When your alarm clock goes off, ACTUALLY GET UP!** Don't linger in bed on social media or your phone for 10-15 minutes. Remember, the more time you spend in bed in the morning, the less time you will have to devote to leisure activities that bring you enjoyment and relaxation.

3.) **Create what I call a "Habit Stack"** routine in the morning. This consists of creating a plan that starts with ONE positive habit early in the day. Then add another positive habit to stack on top of the first until you eventually have a chain of healthy habits. My routine starts with a commitment to ride the bike for 15 minutes as soon as I get up. Afterwards, I stack that with 10 minutes of meditation. It is much easier for our brains to continue on a healthy track once we simply get STARTED. 'Inertia' is now moving in the right direction.

4.) **Eliminate all distractions** from your bedroom that interrupt your sleep patterns. These include televisions, gym equipment, cell phones, iPads, etc., that keep you from winding down at night and reduce the ability for your body to produce melatonin. Melatonin is a hormone integral to the process of inducing sleep. The blue light from these devices (*and yes I know about night mode on the iPhone)* will affect your eyes in such a way that will make it more difficult for you to reach REM sleep. Short for Rapid Eye Movement, REM sleep is the "zone" in which the recovery happens within your body at night. So if it doesn't have to do with sleeping, please remove it from your bedroom immediately!

5.) **Say your prayers before bedtime:** a simple strategy for getting a better night's sleep is to meditate for 5 to 10 minutes while reflecting on what went well during day and what could have been improved. This is a great way to clear your mind from the clutter that might nag at you and keep you awake. Some people keep a notepad in their dresser drawer to write down ideas. This will take away the concern that you might forget them before you drift off to sleep. Sometimes preparing a to-do list for the next day on the notepad can help. Whatever your specific routine, my advice is to keep it simple as you find ways to clear your mind. You'll thank me later.

With these tips for a successful night's sleep, you are equipped with some tangible techniques to improve your life. You may even feel like a new person (a Rockstar!) if you faithfully implement these techniques daily. Your struggle will be building the inertia to implement just one of the changes I listed above. It will take effort and commitment at first, but I promise you, it will be worth it!

Healthy Habit Winning Rule #3: Say your
Prayers and/or Meditate before bed for 10 minutes each night, and watch the quality of your sleep improve drastically.

CHAPTER FOUR

THE BUILDING BLOCKS OF HEALTHY HABITS

Trying something new is not as easy as it sounds, particularly if you are age 50 or above. Why, you may ask? Studies show that after you reach the age of 50, the likelihood that you will deviate from your current habits and patterns is greatly reduced.

Many people in this age group suffer from a lack of curiosity about new activities and ideas. This is due to the fact that your dopamine surge, when you are trying new things later in life, is not as strong as it was in your younger years. Children are naturally curious as they explore and learn all about their environments. Adults lose that curiosity as they age. The good news is our brains are still adaptable and will change through a process called *neuroplasticity*. Case in point - the more you are willing to try new things and explore new ideas (think cultural, political, culinary, travel etc.) the more likely your brain will be to adapt to and actually enjoy change.

Here are some examples of following the same routines, some healthy/ some unhealthy, that plague many of the people I know: dining at the same restaurants every weekend, vacationing at the same location every year, attending the same sporting events/ concerts, getting coffee at the same place every morning, traveling the same route to work each day. You get the drift.

Why do they do it? It is because they tell themselves they are *happy* doing it, but subconsciously the word is *safe*. The same routine is a safe option because you know what the outcome is going to be and you are comfortable with it. You may be happy going to the gym twice a week that you have been a member of for years and riding the bicycle for 20 minutes. You feel safe going to the seafood restaurant near your home because they always serve a decent meal.

What I'm getting at is this: trying anything new causes a slight to moderate uneasy feeling. You consider the following questions. Will this be good for me or not? Will this work for me or not? Will this taste good or not? Will this feel good or not? How will you ever know if you don't push yourself out of your comfort zone?

What can you do to regain a bit of curiosity that might add something different, enjoyable and exciting to your day? I have a few ideas.

Improve your Life by Adding Variety

Have you ever thought about taking a different route to work? Imagine the stores you might drive by that you did not know about, or the new coffee shop or breakfast cafe you could make a plan to try? This would enhance the conversations you have at work while making your day and that of your colleagues a bit more enlightened. Would getting up a few minutes earlier be worth the effort if it meant you were able to learn about new places and see new people?

Time spent in the car is also a great opportunity for self improvement. When you are not passively listening to the radio or chatting with a passenger, you have the opportunity to devote time to an activity that is often understated: Thinking. Many of us fight alone-time as often as possible. Think about our everyday lives. Most of us can balance cooking a meal while talking on the phone and watching the news on TV. Combining these overstimulates the brain. Rarely do we have the opportunity, that is available while riding in the car, to actually *think*. Driving in complete silence is very relaxing. When your body is relaxed you release less of the hormone cortisol, which is known to cause stress and a host of other negative effects on the body.

How many opportunities do you take during the day to experience complete silence or to relax to the sounds of nature? I would venture to guess the answer is "not many." Try stacking on a mini healthy habit by opening a window to capture some fresh air. This will refresh your mind and make you feel a bit better. When driving to work, even in the winter, I typically open the window a crack and take a few deep breaths to help calm my mind as I prepare for the busy day ahead.

When you start asking your brain to 'figure out' new routes to work, or you are consciously using your alone time for self reflection and to pause, your brain will not like it. At least, at first. However your brain's ability to adapt is incredible. All it takes is just a little bit of focus. The brain craves consistency in order to create shortcuts and make the thinking process easier. As you begin, it will be a struggle to convince yourself to take that longer route to work. However, over the course of a week, you will notice it becomes second nature because your brain has already adapted to that path.

Let's stack on to the driving idea. What if you go for a hike in a new town? Or bike in a different park? What if you walk in a neighborhood other than your own? How about taking up golf, swimming or tennis? There are so many options. All you have to do is pick and choose! My dad returned to golf in his 50's after being away from the game for several years. Doing so helped him to meet a host of new people and regain his love for the sport. These are two vital aspects of living a long and healthy life.

Fresh air, new skills, exercise, friendships and a myriad of stories to enrich social conversation resulted from that one decision to resume golfing. You can choose any activity to bring those benefits to your life such as senior center outings, social groups, book clubs, non profit/volunteer clubs. The list goes on, so use your imagination. The possibilities are endless.To give you one piece of advice, I suggest choosing as a *main* hobby, an activity that involves moving. Venture out to join an exercise class or play golf or tennis. Anything that will get you out of the house and into a new social circuit is key.

How to Start a Healthy Habit

Hopefully by now I've got you thinking about starting a new healthy habit. That's excellent! If your habit is something that adds value to your life, you have to make it stick in order for it to last. Let's work with the premise that it takes 21 days to create a habit. That means, if you can maintain a new habit for 3 weeks, chances are that it will become a successful part of your routine.

In his book *Atomic Habits,* author James Clear mentions a few key tips to help you to stay with a habit once you've created it. His first tip, which we have already briefly introduced in this book is called 'habit stacking' and involves stacking your new habit on top of an already existing one. For example, if you are looking to begin a meditation program but struggling to find the time to do so, try the following. Think about the things that you do on a daily basis that are effortless. How about your morning cup of coffee. Simply 'stack' the habit of meditation on to the action of drinking coffee. After you are done with your cup of morning Joe, or while enjoying it, meditate for a set amount of time. Try 10 minutes to start. This will help you create momentum (inertia) based on a habit that you already have to keep you moving in a successful direction.

Small habits can have a surprisingly powerful impact on your life. Imagine a plane taking off from Boston, MA to London, England. If, during takeoff, the pilot decides to adjust his course 3 degrees south, the nose of the plane will move just slightly. Except for the pilots, no one on the plane would notice this small shift. However over the course of the journey across the ocean, the plane may end up as far south as Barcelona, Spain!

Habits Are Like Atoms

It is difficult for us to notice small changes because at first their effect is negligible. Think about trying to lose weight. Taking an hour long walk today, will in all probability not have an effect on the number that will be displayed on the scale when you weigh in tomorrow. However, if you go for an hour long walk everyday for 3 months, you will, in most instances, be leaner and fitter at the end of that time span. The key point is you do not need to revolutionize your behavior. You simply need to make tiny changes to the things that matter most to you. If your health matters, you will make strides to build some of the habits mentioned in this book.

> "Habits are like the atoms of our lives. Each one is a fundamental unit that contributes to your overall improvement." - James Clear

Mind Tricks

Another interesting topic is the relationship of our environment to our ability to make decisions, both positive and negative. Anne Thorndike, a Boston-based doctor, decided to test the following hypothesis. If she set people up to make a better health decision, would they? As part of the test, she had the hospital cafeteria rearranged. Originally the refrigerators near the cash register contained only soft drinks. Thorndike introduced bottled water not only to the checkout line in the cafeteria, but also at every other drink station in the hospital. Over a three month period soft drink sales were down 11% and water sales went up 25%. People just needed the *cue* to drink water. Having water readily available and right in front of them at checkout prompted customers to make better decisions.

Think about your goal of losing weight. What if instead of keeping fruit in the fridge you keep some on the counter? What if you put those tasty crackers that have a prominent spot on your kitchen counter out of sight in the pantry? What if you leave your gym bag and a fresh pair of work clothes in your car? Doing so eliminates the excuse to avoid going to the gym before work in the morning? These are all little environmental cues that will make it easier for you to select healthier choices.

Don't be Vague. Develop a Plan

Most of us say to ourselves, "I want to eat better," but we never end up actually eating better. This is because we do not have a plan to do so. We change our narrative but don't ever follow through because we do not have an implementation strategy in place. Creating a plan can actually be easy. The trick is to start small. A good first step to eating better is "food logging." For instance, you may tell yourself, "I want to eat better, so I'm going to log all of the food I eat during the week in order to determine how many calories I consume each day." This plan is meaningful because it is realistic and is something that will help you understand the scope of where your nutrition habits may be going awry. As a bonus, you get weekends off!

Our brains release dopamine, a hormone that makes us feel good, when we do pleasurable things like eating or procreating. What is often misunderstood is that we also get that same dose of dopamine by just anticipating pleasurable events! Desiring something is on a par with actually receiving something. Think about the vacation you had looked forward to for a long time. I'm sure the vacation was great. But was the vacation really all it was cracked up to be? Or was the sense of anticipation what you really enjoyed? How can you use the principal of dopamine release to improve your ability to live a healthier lifestyle? Try combining something you love, eating, with something you don't enjoy, perhaps exercise. Then after you work out, reward yourself with the steak you have been salivating over all day. How can you apply this approach to your love for watching a midday SOAP opera? I suggest that during the episode, you ride on a recumbent bike at a sub-maximal effort. This way, you are able to accomplish your daily calorie burn by riding the bike while getting your dopamine kick from catching up on the latest plot line from your favorite show.

How to Make it Easy to Build a New Habit

Let's discuss the concept of *friction*- specifically in terms of how friction can help us create good habits while steering us away from bad ones. As an example, my staff is much more likely to send thank-you cards to someone who refers a friend or family member if the cards are readily available at the front desk at all times. There is minimal friction in this interaction because all the staff member needs to do is take a card, which is in plain sight, and write the message. However, if the thank-you cards are hidden in a drawer in my office, what are the chances that anyone would ever receive a card from my office? Probably pretty slim. Hopefully this helps you to understand the concept of creating or reducing friction related to a behavior. The circumstances you create will either make it an easier or more difficult habit to adopt. To equate this to your desire to exercise and lose weight, simply keep that shiny new spin bike right by your bedside. Then when you wake up in the morning you know what your first task is: to ride the bike.

Another example of creating friction is to unplug your television after watching it. This will make it that much more difficult to sit down and 'veg' in front of the TV for hours. If it is not as easy as simply pressing the power button on the remote, you will be less likely to perform the activity- in this case watching TV.

Another trick for making a habit easier in the long term is sticking to something called the two-minute rule. Simplify a task into something that can be done in two minutes or less. For instance, if you want to learn how to garden in retirement, commit 2 minutes each day to reading a gardening book. Chances are that you will probably spend more than 2 minutes reading. If you commit to the activity and make it easy you are more likely to achieve it.

A final and most important rule is to make your newfound 'healthy habits' satisfying. This phenomenon of satisfaction can be a tricky one, especially in the immediate gratification-environment in which we live. Think how long it takes to achieve satisfaction from losing 10 pounds! We are wired to want immediate results in all aspects of life. So when you are looking to pursue habits with a delayed return, try to attach some immediate gratification to them. Let's say you and your partner are hoping to eat healthier and save money from eating out. Each time you cook dinner at home, instead of going out to eat, put the $100 you would have spent on dining out into an account named "trip to the Caribbean." This way you have the satisfaction of saving for your beach trip as an immediate reward for cooking at home. You have had a healthy meal and saved money.

Quality Thinking Time

Who do you spend the most time with? Your spouse? Your dog? Your children? Think again! It's YOU! What an opportunity this provides for meditation. The benefits of meditation are well known and have an affect on many aspects of life. Some of the benefits of meditation that we currently know are:

- Improved mood
- Improved focus and decreased 'mind wandering'
- Decreased Anxiety/ Agitation/ Depression
- Improved Self- Compassion
- Reduced stress including reduction in Systolic BP

... and those are just a few. Now imagine if you are able to incorporate any of these benefits into your life and how your life might look in 1 week, 1 month and 1 year? Who wouldn't want to have more focus and improved mood well into old age? I certainly would.

Here's the trick.

Start by dedicating just *10 minutes a day* to mindfulness. These 10 minutes can be spent in your house, office, favorite park, or anywhere you are comfortable. The key ingredient is that you are ALONE with your thoughts with absolutely NO DISTRACTIONS. Our brains need to unwind and rest in order to function properly. That is part of the reason why we require REM sleep at night - to recover properly. When you meditate, a wonderful thing happens. The world stops. You are able to be in the present moment, where study after study continues to prove is the place we are most fulfilled, and recognize the moment for what it is. Maybe you have aches and pains, or social or emotional issues that are vexing you. This is the time of the day where you recognize these issues, acknowledge their presence, put them aside, and move forward to focus on what you are grateful for and why life is worth living. Meditation can be a great healer.

CHAPTER FIVE

HOW TO LIVE A HAPPIER LIFE

How do we live happier lives? When we take the time to write out what we are grateful for, it almost always requires us to pause for a moment to think about what is pursuant to family, friends, and your relationship to God (if you are religious). The old saying is, "you never truly appreciate what you have until it's gone." Imagine losing everything: your possessions, your friends, loved ones, your health and independence. Next imagine slowly getting each of those back one at a time. How grateful would you be?

You shouldn't have to lose things that matter in order to be grateful for them. Unfortunately, most of us are consistently in a state of reaction. Instead of being grateful for all of the positivity in our lives, we react to anything that may bring harm to our way of life. Gratitude is tied directly to happiness. Many people take their health and independence for granted. As both a PT and a business owner, I see this all too often. Do they truly appreciate getting in and out of their "retirement sports car," spending a weekend hiking with their grandchildren on mount Monadnock, or any of the other activities they enjoy? The answer for most is probably not. That is, not until those activities are put on hold for a week, month, or even as long as 365 days. It can take up to one year to recover from spinal fusion surgery or a joint replacement. My point is to appreciate what you have today because tomorrow it could be gone!

You have the most control over your own happiness. Instead of external pursuits and seeking happiness from material belongings, my suggestion is to look within. What can you change about your perspective to enjoy life more today?

Long term happiness does not come from things which we cannot control- the stock market, jobs, relationships, or life-changing events good or bad. Happiness is grounded in what you are able to control, namely your perspective on the world and your relationship to everything in it. My two principles of happiness are:

1. You must stay grounded in the present
2. You must have a positive outlook on the world

By focusing on well-being and personal fulfillment (instead of wealth and power, for instance) you will be well on your way to living a healthier life. Fortunately, wherever you are on your journey, it is relatively easy to focus on well-being and personal fulfillment. Choose just one or two activities you love, then make sure you practice them on a weekly basis. You might take pleasure in going to church, traveling, gardening, or playing tennis or pickle-ball. Whatever your hobby is, choose something and stick to it! Block out time for your favorite hobby by putting it on your schedule and guarding it with your life. As an example,

I time block my Tuesday afternoons for golf. Golfing allows me to enjoy the outdoors and clear my head. It gives me a fresh perspective on patient care and business goals that I may never have thought of if I stayed in the office all day.

We all have one or two things we love to do. Amazingly, the hard part is putting our passion into practice in order to improve our lives. Like any habit, the longer we stay with something the better the effect. Allow 60-70 days to not only form, but to solidify your habit. I encourage you to take my advice, go out, and enjoy life a little bit. You never know what a fresh perspective and gratitude may do for your personal well-being.

How to Instill a Healthy Habit in Just 21 Days

How much time do you *think* you spend on daily mundane tasks. A great way to find out how much you spend watching television, checking your smartphone, looking at facebook/ instagram/ twitter etc. is to begin to log the amount of time. Your smartphone may already do this on its own. Do this each day for (3) days. Record the time you spend performing your daily tasks. This is a technique that is a commodity in "Self-Help" books- *just write down everything you do for a week and then look at all the time you could allocate to other endeavors!*

We have all heard that suggestion. The question is: Who can actually follow through and put this technique into practice? I promise you will be astounded by the outcome of this exercise.

> **Healthy Habit Winning Rule #4:** Log the time you spend on any activity for (3) straight days. Then carefully analyze what you can eliminate to make more time in your day.

New Beginnings and New Habits

Have you ever tried to change a bad habit, like leaving the toilet seat up or eating junk food? It is not easy. I think we've already established that! Part of the reason why it is so difficult to change our habits is because our daily routines play a strong role in controlling our behavior. So the question is: How do we interrupt that feedback loop so that we can move out of *stasis* and into *positive inertia?* How do we hit the 'reset' button in order to change the regularity that is built into our daily lives? Routines are ingrained at a neural level to make our brain's job easier. Our brains are wired to find shortcuts and loathe the long way around! Our bodies love regularity. If we are unhappy with some of our habits, a great way to change is to find your version of a *new beginning.*

Let me explain what I mean. A new beginning commonly occurs with a major life shift. For example, moving to a new city, town or province is a classic new beginning. Other examples include starting a new job, a new relationship, a new company, a new book, a new friendship, a new hobby. You get the point. A new beginning is a great way to interrupt the neural feedback loop that your body is comfortable with.

Consider a study of people who wanted to improve their diet by eating healthier. More than 36% of participants were successful with their new diets when they moved to a new location. Why is that? Part of the reason for success in staying with a new habit is the dopamine rush (what makes your brain and body feel happy) received when you are acclimating to a new environment. Couple, or stack, that experience with something that you have been wanting to do and you begin to see results. WHAM, you've got a winning dopamine release combination!

The point is to try something new when you are older. Do not give up. For instance, now that you are retired, why not try that Pilates or Barre class you have always been thinking about? This is a way to bank on the infusion of dopamine resulting from a new activity. One that will contribute to your overall well-being and life satisfaction.

Healthy Habit Winning Rule #5: Try something new that you have been hesitant to do before. Your brain will reward you for it.

Start Framing Any Movement as Exercise

A common lament I hear in my clinic is, "Dr. Lordan, I just hate to exercise!" (I could have used a more subtle word than hate.) This mindset is pervasive among many people. I would prefer not to admit it. The truth is that we are wired to do the bare minimum necessary to survive. Exercise is an activity that is commonly made out to be a boring, energy laden task that few of us like to make time for in our busy day- to-day lives. Everyone is familiar with the extensive benefits of exercise, so why is it that just 23% of us get the exercise we need? Only 1 in 10 Americans pay a monthly subscription to go to a gym. No wonder there is an obesity epidemic in the United States!

For the purposes of this section we will shy away from how adiposity affects the lives of millions of Americans in a negative way, and instead focus on why so many of us dislike exercise. My belief is that as a society we are simply lazy. It requires much less effort to sit on the couch and binge watch Netflix than it does to get up and go to the Pilates class across town. I understand this. I hear this nearly every day. So what can you do about it? For starters, you need to reframe the way you think about exercise and turn it into an activity that is simple. Exercise by definition is movement or activity that requires physical exertion or effort. Can you think of something in your life that requires physical effort or exertion that you actually like to do? Great! Start with that.

Getting enough exercise is really easy, yet most people don't know where to start. I understand how performing basic physical exercises can be boring and cumbersome, but as a PT, I do try to make them fun! You can too. Going to the gym and doing 3 sets of 10 repetitions of leg presses, dumbbell-curls, and squats can be boring and time consuming for some.

Let me enlighten you. Going for a half hour walk with your dog is just as beneficial as walking on the treadmill at a slight incline for 20 minutes.The key is to simply get out and move. Outdoor activities are excellent because fresh air has a way of stimulating our senses to maximize the benefits of the activity. Our brains and intrinsic motivations begin to shift and crave this daily walk or bike ride. As a result, our metabolisms slowly start to change.

Walking up and down stairs a few times a day to do a couple loads of laundry is another great exercise. Taking a loop around a neighborhood, preferably in a new part of town, will maximize the novelty and dopamine/endorphin rush! Going for a High Intensity Interval Workout at your local Gym or *Orange Theory* may be your preference. What is most important is identifying the way you prefer to move to begin capitalizing on the benefits of exercise. Experiencing aches and pains when you introduce exercise into your daily routine, is to be expected with the normal aging process. With proper technique and consistency, this will be temporary. If the discomfort begins to rate above a 5 on a scale of 1-10 (10 being the worst imaginable pain) or is sharp or burning in nature, then you should contact a medical professional for a proper workup. In subsequent chapters, I will discuss specifically how to rehab some of the common ailments associated with aging. In general, look out for the following red flags. If any are present during or after a workout, please reach out to your Primary Care or Physical Therapist as soon as possible.

- Sharp pain that is persistent in nature
- Burning pain, or shooting sensations in your legs and feet
- An audible "pop" or "snap"
- Bruised muscles after a workout
- Trouble catching your breath or experiencing lightheadedness

CHAPTER SIX

NAVIGATING YOUR GOLDEN YEARS

Retirement is a wonderful time of life. Hopefully, a time for reflection and enjoyment of leisure activities. Although many plan for retirement, a large number of people are forced into early retirement due to poor health and lifestyle choices. More than one third of Americans reported in 2017 that health was a 'very important factor' for their retirement.

Who does not want to be able to live out their glory years in comfort with good health? After all, you have earned it! There are some caveats that I would like to touch upon and discuss concerning retirement.

Retirement offers the opportunity for an individual to reconnect with family, friends and hobbies. So many things that were important to them throughout their lives, but were never a priority due to other pressing tasks (raising a family, work, religious obligations, etc.) Pre-retirement daily lives are often packed with transporting children to soccer games, working long hours, volunteering at a community event or simply doing a myriad of things that need to get done. As a new retiree it is important to realize that you now have the ability to reinvest that time. Start reaping the dividends of having time available to invest in yourself. Do not take for granted a moment of the time you have left on earth.

Best Health Tips for Retirement

In order to realize your retirement dream, it is important that you perform a few tasks everyday that will help you live a healthy lifestyle well into your 80's and 90's. There is one specific tip that I firmly believe will help you live a better life today: create a daily stretching routine. If I had a quarter for every 65+ year old client whose chief complaint was "muscle stiffness/ muscle aches," I would be a very rich man. The easiest way to combat everyday muscle aches and pains is to stretch! A simple **daily** routine with the following three steps will get you started:

1. Perform 10 Cook Squats
2. Perform a prayer stretch for 1 minute
3. Perform a calf stretch while standing on a step for 1 minute

Notice that I stressed the word daily. The key for stretching properly and getting lasting results is to make sure that you stretch consistently over a long period of time. It is important to be consistent because your tissues will respond to improved muscle length only if they are challenged on a daily basis. 3-4 times a week is not enough. This advice differs from the traditional work-out mindset that your muscles generally need time to recover and will grow during the off days. Unfortunately, if you don't stretch everyday you will likely start to live with those nasty aches and pains that you have vehemently tried to avoid.

Health Opportunities in Retirement

When you retire the world is your oyster and opportunity abounds. Many choose to use retirement to "relax", catch up on books, watch television shows that they have missed out on during their working years, and other sedentary activities. However, you need to move. Looking in the classifieds as discussed earlier, you will find plenty of activities for you to go out and get involved in. New activities will help both your brain and body grow. They will renew an old sense of vitality (again back to that good old fashioned dopamine rush!) My challenge for you is to spend two minutes picturing what you want your life to look like. What is your dream life? Are you on a boat in the Caribbean or skiing in the Alps? Whatever it is, take steps to make this dream become reality. Part of the reason you retire is to pursue you dreams. Remember, you only live once! Go out and travel the world now that your children are off to school or out on their own. The more activities that you engage in, the more likely you will be to stick to the healthy habits that are allowing you to perform at your best in the first place.

Is Age Really Just a Number?

One of my favorite questions from clients is: "Am I too old to be doing this?"

What a question this is. There are many answers and only a handful of healthcare providers will be completely honest with you regarding what your activity limit should be as you age (frankly because they are unsure). The conventional medical model rewards playing it safe when it comes to exercising and recreation as we age. If you are 60 or older, I suggest that you consult your Primary Care Doctor to make sure that you are healthy enough to begin a training and recreation program. Most of the time during your annual appointment, your physician will review the list of medications you are currently taking, gauge your blood pressure and heart rate, and do a mild exercise test. In some cases they may perform a "stress test." Generally, however, as healthcare providers, we just want to know that your heart and blood vessels can handle the increased pressure to the system that comes with working out or playing tennis. Be sure to have a checkup, similar to the aforementioned, if you have ever felt short of breath walking up a flight of stairs, or when taking a long walk.

Reduce the Age You Feel in Seven Steps

Is age really just a number? I believe you are as old as you *feel*. I have met 60 year olds who are able to perform personal bests consistently at CrossFit due to an uncommonly high level of self control and diligence when it comes to their nutrition and stretching routines. I have also come across sexagenarians who cannot bend over to tie their shoes, and others who have to use a walker or cane often due to poor lifestyle choices, sometimes only made within the past 5 years. Of course genetics will play some role in who you are physically. What you become can be modified by what we in the biz call "Lifestyle Variables." These help you to "cheat" the system by making you look and feel younger than you really are. The following are 7 main lifestyle habits that contribute to how old you REALLY are.

1. Exercise Habits
2. Stress Levels
3. Nutritional Habits
4. Level of Education
5. Alcohol / Nicotine Consumption
6. Amount of Sleep
7. Sexual and Romantic Relationships

Now that you know the main contributing variables to your biological age, I will talk a little bit about addressing each topic individually to create some lasting changes. The most important suggestion that I will repeat throughout this book is to simply take this one step at a time. Many of us will get overwhelmed trying to implement everything overnight, but recall it takes 21 days on average to create a habit **and approximately 66 days to solidify it.** So please take it easy on yourself and do not bite off more than you can chew. Start with 2 things and implement a small change over the course of 2 months. I call this the 2x2 rule. For example, you can commit to eliminating all alcohol from your diet and to getting 8 hours of sleep every night for 2 months. Keep a journal to track your progress and see how it goes. If you are unable to successfully manage this that's OK- the point is you tried. It is however important to start with something you know you will be successful at and build from there, as we discussed earlier. This will build inertia and allow you to experience a healthy and fulfilling retirement.

Healthy Habit Winning Rule #6: Start small and follow the 2x2 rule. Start with 2 positive habits and implement a small change over the course of 2 months.

7 Steps You Can Adopt TODAY to Feel Physically and Mentally Younger:

1. Stop smoking and drinking alcohol
2. Add more fruits, vegetables, lean meats and water to your diet
3. Create more intimacy with your partner and invest more time in your closest relationships
4. Practice good sleep patterns by eliminating screens and relaxing for an hour before you go to sleep
5. Start a walking or exercise program
6. Practice mindfulness
7. Try intermittent fasting, eating within an 8 hour window each day and keeping the timing consistent (10am - 6pm for example)

There you have it: 7 secrets to reduce the age you feel and contribute to a happier life well into your 80's and 90's.

CHAPTER SEVEN

KNEE TIPS TO KEEP THE DOCTOR AWAY

Janice O. aged 55 once asked me, "Dr. Lordan, every time I'm walking on the beach or around town in sandals for a long time, my feet, knees and low back are killing me afterwards. Do I have plantar fasciitis? Is it arthritis? Is it my footwear? Am I doing something wrong? I feel like I can't enjoy the simple activities I used to love like cooking dinner for my family or going for walks with my friends. Can you help?"

Gravity Always Prevails

A common fact is that as we age our bodies change. One of the truths of aging is that gravity will always prevail! This means that joints become more congruent, the act of joint surfaces coming closer over time, due to what we in the medical profession call *approximation*. The cause of approximation is gravity related, although with a healthy exercise regiment and nutrition routine, you can mitigate the effects of gravity by training the extensor muscle groups in your body. I will delve into training techniques later in this chapter.

It is important that we touch on the effects of aging on our knees and other joints. Aging causes degeneration of the joints. Most physicians and medical professionals will argue that this is just a fact of life. I am never surprised when a septuagenarian client brings in an X-Ray showing degenerative changes in the knees. In fact the radiologist usually writes in the impression: *normal age-related degeneration of the joint presents at the Tibial Plateau/ Femoral Condyles.... etc.* The fact that degeneration of the cartilage is present is not the root cause of the knee pain. Many older adults experience cartilaginous changes and for the most part are asymptomatic with the exception of a few snaps, crackles, and pops here and there. The question is: can exercise fix it or do you need surgery?

Is Surgery Necessary?

Degenerative Joint Disease (DJD) is a fact of aging. What can be done to beat it? The answer is exercise. Studies show time after time that those who live a more active lifestyle by getting the CDC's (Center for Disease Control) recommended allotment of weekly exercise, will have less joint pain as they age. Listed below are the 2020 CDC guidelines regarding exercise.

150 minutes of moderate intensity aerobic exercise (walking, hiking or working an active job requiring you to be on your feet)

-OR-

75 minutes of vigorous physical activity: (Pilates or Yoga class, High Intensity Interval Training, Running)

You do not need a fancy gym membership to exercise. The bottom line is the more you move the better you feel. This leads me into the next Healthy Habit Winning Rule.

Healthy Habit Winning Rule #7: Perform a 30 minute walk or bike ride, or workout vigorously twice a week for 45 minutes.

If you can adopt winning rule number 7 your chances for staving off knee pain in the foreseeable future will be more promising.

Why Does the Weather Bother my Joints?

In New England, we like to refer to the months of November, December, January, and February as the "doldrums" of the year! Typically most of us (yes, myself included!) suffer from seasonal affective disorder (SAD). We do not get enough Vitamin D from sunlight and are consequently in a funk. It is difficult to elevate our moods due to the frigid temperatures and a decrease in the amount of daylight hours. Both of these affect our joints and bodies in other deleterious ways too.

During cold weather, your blood flows from its extremities inward to keep your vital organs warm. The subsequent reduction in blood flow leaves fewer white blood cells to fight disease. Bacteria and viruses brew increasing your risk for catching the "Common Cold." It's called "a Cold" for a reason! Who knew?

There is controversy over the reason why cold weather makes our joints ache, especially as we age. There is no simple explanation for why dropping temperatures affect your joints.

Some theorize that a drop in barometric pressure can cause tendons, muscles and the surrounding tissues to expand. This can result in confined space causing pain, especially in joints affected by arthritis.

Others theorize that when the cartilage that covers the bone surfaces wears away over time (DJD), the nervous system receptors on the bony surface may react to the barometric pressure changes, resulting in pain and inflammation.

Winter weather also brings about the tendency to 'hibernate.' Many of us look forward to this time of year, spending evenings reading a book under a warm blanket in lieu of going for a walk around the neighborhood. However, this decrease in overall activity indicates a higher likelihood that joints will become stiff and painful.

There is an antidote: Movement! All you have to do to combat winter's onslaught is simply get in your car and drive to the gym. If a gym is not accessible to you, try going up and down a set of stairs 10 times, or exercise to a workout video from YouTUBE on your television. There are really no excuses not to move. Do not give in!

Achy Knees, What Not to Do

If you have had achy knees for a while and are not sure what you should do, ask yourself: Should I call my doctor (PCP)? Should I go straight to a specialist? Would I benefit from seeing a physical therapist? All good questions. In most states you can by-pass your PCP and seek the advice of a PT who will evaluate your situation. Most insurances will cover an evaluation and follow-up visits, if needed.

My first question to you would be: *How do you rate your pain?* If you have been limping for a while but your pain is under control (think < 5 on a scale of 1-10; 10 being Emergency Room level pain), I would suggest that you go straight to your local PT office. If your pain is excruciating (>8/10), I recommend going to the ER or local Urgent Care to have imaging done, (X-Ray/ MRI) etc., to make sure there isn't an underlying fracture or infection. Typically your PCP will take an X-Ray at a yearly physical if you are complaining of slight knee pain to rule out anything more serious than arthritis or DJD diagnosis. My next question is: *Then what?*

Typically the questions that I am asked by a client at the initial PT examination are: Should I be wearing a brace? If so, what kind of brace? Should I buy CBD oil or use BenGay/ BioFreeze? What about Ice/ Heat- which one is better? Should I be taking ibuprofen? Do I need a cortisone shot? Do I need surgery? What about Synvisk injections? The list goes on and on! Let me address a few of these topics to inform you about the basics.

Brace? Good or Bad?

Please do not put on a knee brace without first consulting a physical therapist to determine if one is actually needed, and, if so, which one is best for you. Many times NO BRACE is necessary. The reason being, when you use an external support to help stabilize your knee joint, your muscles and ligaments *do less work*. When your muscles and ligaments are supported, thereby performing less work, they can atrophy or decay. This muscle weakness is the prime reason for your knee pain in the first place. Often, using a knee brace makes your knee pain worse.

Barring an underlying joint instability like ligamentous insufficiency or patella dislocation, avoid bracing at all costs.

Joint Creams and Rubs

Many folks enjoy the short term benefits of using joint sprays and creams to help ameliorate the symptoms of joint pain. The knee is a common site of joint pain and as such is a typical site of application of creams and rubs. My advice is to look into what you are putting on your body and consult with your PCP or local pharmacist to make sure that it is safe and FDA approved. The process of FDA approval is highly regulated. Beware, many substandard products are available but with major risks. The companies producing those do not spend the necessary time or money on being properly vetted. As a result, products that are not FDA approved *do not need to list the proper amounts of active ingredients used* and may be unsafe for public consumption. I recommend opting for brands that have been around for a long time. The way many of these creams work is similar. Most contain menthol and/or methyl salicylate, known joint counterirritants. They work by causing the skin to feel cool and then warm, which "tricks" your nervous system into a feeling of hypoalgesia (less pain sensation). Essentially they act as a "distraction," offering temporary relief, and are not the answer to eliminating the aches and pains from arthritis.

Ice or Heat?

The ultimate rehab question and the one most commonly asked of my staff and me is: "Which is better, Ice or Heat?" The answer depends on a multiplicity of variables. I will break it down into common instances that I professionally use for each.

When to Ice

If your joints are swollen, achy or painful and it is toward the END of the day, use an ice pack to help control the swelling and inflammation. Ice reduces tissue temperature, thereby decreasing cellular metabolism in the injured area. This helps decrease the inflammatory cascade by slowing the process down to help mitigate further inflammation. Ice is best used in the minutes immediately after an injury. This is a time when it is important to follow the PRICE protocol: Pressure, Rest, Ice, Compression, Elevation. For example, if you twist your knee, hear a pop or just feel something funny in your knee while you are walking, and if it begins to swell, elevate the joint above heart level and apply ice by wrapping the ice around the knee.

When to Heat

First of all, the type of 'Heat' matters. At our clinic, we use moist heat which is the best way to deliver heat to muscles and joints due to its controlled release of heat over time. Some over the counter variants of hot packs require you to boil or microwave them. Beware that these products will burn you if you are not careful! Now that the safety box is checked, I will begin with this admonishment: **Do NOT apply heat immediately after an injury!** This is the worst time to use heat because it will accelerate the inflammatory cascade and make your pain worse.

I advise clients to heat their joints in the morning via a hot shower or by applying a hot pack to the affected joint. This will help them to get the day started well by loosening up their muscles and joints. Heat has a way of decreasing muscle tension and improving pliability. Adding heat to muscles will soothe 'charley horses' and muscle aches by increasing vasodilation (blood-flow) to the area promoting improved circulation. It is key to understand that during an ACUTE injury, you do not want more circulation! Heat should be used sparingly in the weeks immediately after a total joint replacement or surgery. It should be directed toward the post operative muscle groups around the joint being worked on, not on the joint itself.

Are Cortisone Shots Helpful?

Simply put, yes they can be. Depending on the amount of inflammation present in the knee combined with your pain level, cortisone shots do well getting your symptoms under control so that you can tolerate an exercise program. Please do not be fooled here. A cortisone shot will not fix your knee pain problem. A recent study (October 2017) out of the *National Institute of Arthritis and Musculoskeletal and Skin Diseases revealed* that folks who received cortisone shots repeatedly over a 2 year period had no long-term pain relief compared to those who received a placebo. The injections actually sped up the process of cartilage deterioration, a well known common side effect of repeat corticosteroid injection. So please seek out the care of a physical therapist to address your knee pain as a first step. You won't regret it!

Do I Need Foot Inserts?

Now let's tackle the topic of foot inserts. These have many names and are readily available in your local pharmacy aisle touting a "free test, step here" fitting process where-by a machine delineates the perfect D*r. Scholl's* foot insert for you or your loved one. My personal opinion, and one backed by science as well, is that over the counter (OTC) orthotics are pricey and not worth it. If you have pain in your feet, or you spend a lot of time standing throughout the course of the day, then a consult with a podiatrist or physical therapist is a first step in determining which type of foot insert (if any) will be helpful.

Two Main Types of Professional Orthotics

Without going too far in depth, it is important to note that there are two main types of orthotic inserts for the feet. The first type is called "semi-rigid". Semi-rigid orthotic devices are used to control motion of a hyper-mobile foot. The insert is made of a hard plastic (semi-rigid) material that sits underneath the arch and supports the foot throughout the stance phase of gait. Common diagnoses that benefit from a semi-rigid orthotic device include plantar fasciitis, patella-femoral pain syndrome, ITB syndrome and shin splints. The second type of orthotic is a "semi-flexible" device. A semi-flexible orthotic is typically made of a more cushioned cork material that has some "give." This type is designed to alleviate pain for the wearer. Those who experience arthritis or who are older tend to benefit from the semi-flexible devices. These orthotics are less invasive to the natural structure of the foot and are thus tolerated much better by a wearer with a sensitive foot structure or one of advanced age.

The key to a proper orthotic prescription is a skilled assessment of the lower body and gait mechanics. Because of the many nuances that pertain to which type of orthotic is best, the assessment is crucial. There are details to consider including what material to use for the arch, what to cover the device with, and whether modifications are needed for decreased toe or metatarsal range of motion. It is also important that the factory where the orthotics are made is owned and operated by a certified orthotist, most of whom have a master's or doctorate degree in the field of orthotics and prosthetics. My advice is to find a practitioner whom you trust. Orthotics can be very expensive and may not work for you. Seek a provider who will use the right combination of materials and make sure you have a proper fit!

How to Improve Knee Pain Without Painkillers

The effects of the opioid epidemic on patients with knee osteoarthritis are severe. Excessive opioid use in patients leads to poorer patient satisfactions as well as increased morbidities and mortalities. Many folks turn to narcotic and non-narcotic medications alike to alleviate symptoms associated with chronic knee pain. The problem with medication is that it does not get to the root cause of the problem. If you have a meniscus tear, for instance, taking a pain pill will do nothing to fix the symptoms associated with that tear. However, with a proper strength and stretching regimen, and potentially hands-on therapy, knee pain will generally become less severe in just a matter of weeks. Additionally, the use of a custom insert in your shoes will significantly improve knee pain caused by OA, patella-femoral pain syndrome, and for those with hyper-pronated feet.

There are many exercises that you can perform to help lessen knee pain and prevent it from returning. In the appendix of the book, you will find an album of exercises to help improve your knee strength and mobility safety that we commonly perform at my clinic. You can also go to conciergephysicaltherapy.com/-knee-pain-free-report to learn 7 very effective principles and strategies you can incorporate into your lifestyle, for short-term and long-term success. These techniques are used to treat knee pain at Concierge PT.

CHAPTER EIGHT

FOR THOSE STRUGGLING WITH LOW BACK PAIN: SOME RELIEF

Who Gets Low Back Pain and Why?

Low back pain (LBP) is one of the most prevalent medical conditions in the world. As many as 1 in 3 people will be afflicted with LBP this year for the first time. LBP is the leading cause of activity limitation and absence from work throughout the world and is associated with an enormous economic burden. For those who have experienced LBP early in life, there is a 33% reoccurrence rate during later years. In general, women are more likely than men to have low back pain, and older folks are more likely to have debilitating LBP. Unfortunately, those without a high school diploma are at a higher risk of LBP and typically have a longer episode duration and worse clinical outcomes. So what can you do today to avoid becoming a statistic tomorrow? Read further and find out!

Dad Had LBP, am I Doomed?

Many variables determine your likelihood of acquiring LBP throughout the course of your life. Included among those determinants are: genetics, age, gender, build, strength and flexibility. Specific disorders of the spine including those surrounding degeneration have strong genetic links. So yes, if your father or mother has had severe degenerative changes to their spine, then you are at an increased risk for the same.

The development of non-specific LBP is shrouded in a bit more mystery. Non-specific LBP refers to pain in the lower back region that is not attributable to any specific pathology, such as herniated disc, cancer, tumor or degeneration. Unfortunately, degenerative changes shown on an MRI or other medical scan do not correlate well to pain level. Many folks have scans showing these changes of the spine and show no symptoms at all; while others may have mild degenerative symptoms and can barely walk due to pain and numbness emanating from the spine. Spinal imaging is not an accurate indicator of the root cause of LBP symptoms. A clinician must perform a comprehensive physical exam in order to determine what impairments are contributing factors. Typically the root cause is a combination of some of the following: tight and weak muscles, poor diet, inadequate hydration, decreased activity, job requiring heavy-lifting, history of injury and avoidance of moving due to fear of moving the wrong way.

Why Rest is the Worst Thing You Can Do

There is a consistent relationship in the literature that compares outcomes of those who are sedentary immediately after "throwing out their backs" and those who are less fearful of moving. Those who move right away do better. Fear is an instinct that is a natural part of our brains primal protection process. In the case of LBP, fear causes us to refrain from movement because we think it will cause more pain. However, those who don't move and stay bedridden for a week or two after an acute mechanical back injury are at a much higher risk for chronic pain and debility, both short and long term. Your back craves motion. Since the spinal discs get their nutrition through osmosis, not through blood vessels unless there is damage to the disc, the healing process can take much longer. However, it is aided by gentle movements. In the appendix, I have provided several movements that I highly recommend for the phases immediately following an acute back injury (fractures excluded). Fractures and post operative cases are a bit more complicated because the body needs time to heal. Generally, though, the premise is the same. Your spine is the key to movement throughout your body. If your spine is not performing well, every joint will experience a taxing effect.

Do I Need to See a Primary Care Doctor First?

Another question that I am often asked is: "Do I need to go to my Primary Care Physician (PCP) before I come to see you?" The answer is, it depends. In Massachusetts, and many other states as well, you are able to see a physical therapist first through what is called 'Direct Access.' Direct Access means that by law you are allowed to be evaluated by a PT without having to schedule an appointment with your PCP. Whether your insurance will cover this depends on your plan. Many do. Seeing a PT first allows your PT to "Quarterback" your healthcare and determine whether you need an X-Ray, an MRI, a cortisone shot or PRP injection. You may not. In my humble opinion, I think this is the best path for any musculoskeletal injury. Research shows that PTs are on par with orthopedic surgeons when it comes to accurately diagnosing musculoskeletal injuries, when compared to MRI results.

The cost of care is, on average, 50% less if you go to a PT directly versus going through your PCP or orthopedic doctor. Unnecessary tests and measures are often over prescribed prior to PT intervention. A hands-on therapeutic approach will yield the same, if not better, outcomes. My advice is to call your insurance agent to find out what your benefits and eligibility are prior to planning any visits to a doctor. Most people are not educated about the benefits available on their plans. Call your insurance representative who will guide and inform you. But, bear in mind, it is your job to seek out the local experts to solve your problems, not theirs! The bottom line is you will most likely save money and a lot of hassle if you see a PT first.

What Should I Try Before Asking for Help

I implore those who experience low back pain for the first time to rest and apply ice for the first 48 hours, in 20 minute intervals. After that it is imperative that you get your body moving in a safe manner. Depending on how the back pain occurred, movement will be based on a direction that will restore motion lost in a safe way. NSAIDs help in the acute phase of an injury, but can also contribute to a delay in healing per some recent post surgical studies. My advice is to refer to the exercises in the appendix. They will help guide you through the phases of general low back rehab. The goals of initial therapy are to reduce pain levels and restore motion. Strength comes with time, which is why it is so important to have a strong core to begin with, considering the aging process works against you. You may lose up to one percent of muscle tissue per year after age 35 due to sarcopenia, but again, with proper training the effects of muscular atrophy associated with aging can be negated.

What Are the Best Exercises for Low Back Pain

When it comes to exercise prescriptions for low back pain, there is no "one size fits all" approach. Evidence strongly suggests that a moderate to intense graded exercise regimen will significantly improve chronic low back pain. It is important to understand that if you are experiencing significant amounts of pain you should call your PCP or PT directly to go over the best exercise strategy to get started. There are three main phases of the rehab process. In each phase the exercises differ.

Acute Phase (Week 0-4)

During the acute phase of a LBP problem, many are unable to move in certain directions and fear making the pain worse. In this stage it is imperative to do gentle exercises to get the spine moving again and to limit the inflammation from increasing. Many times medications like Flexeril and Ibuprofen are adjuncts that will help in the first few days of a LBP attack. As an aside, let me also be clear that if you are having trouble with your bowel or bladder, or are experiencing "saddle numbness" or decreased peritoneal sensation, please go to an urgent care or ER immediately.

Some may use opiates in this phase due to the severe pain involved. I caution against this. Opiates do not target the pain at the location of the infarct, but rather in the brain, and are very addictive. Opiates also potentially mask the severity of an injury and may allow you to move into positions that your body would normally guard against to prevent further debilitation. This phase of exercises and treatment should consist of some gentle pelvic tilts, lower trunk rotations and gluteus activation. If severe pain persists any longer than 3 days, my advice is to visit a local urgent care center or your PCP office to get basic imaging to help define the patho-anatomics of the problem before it gets worse.

Subacute Phase (Weeks 4-12)

The subacute phase occurs when the body begins to strengthen the exercise foundation built upon during the acute phase of recovery. Generally speaking it takes 6-8 weeks to increase muscle strength as a function of hypertrophy and power. During this phase you will build on either a directional approach or a neutral spine approach. I will include both flexion and extension exercises in the appendix. Depending on your diagnosis, age, prior medical history and gender your exercise approach will vary in this stage of recovery.

If you are a 40 year old male with no past medical history and have had a disc herniation, try McKenzie extension exercises. If you are a 65 year old female with a history of DDD (degenerative disc disease) and spondylolisthesis, try a flexion based approach. My advice is to start with the "neutral spine" exercises in the appendix and build on those with a directional preference: Flexion or Extension. Here are a few diagnoses with which you will want to try the Flexion approach first: DDD, DJD, Stenosis, Arthritis, Spondyloarthropathy, Spondylolysis, Spondylolisthesis. Conversely, if you have one of these diagnoses try extension first: Disc Herniation, Chronic LBP, Sciatica, Numbness and Tingling in either lower extremity. If you are uncertain of the diagnosis, the safest approach is to start with a neutral spine approach. If you don't notice any change or are tending to experience more pain, reach out to your local PT.

Chronic Stage (Weeks 12+)

This stage tends to be aligned with increased ratings of depression and fear of movement. Both of these are negatively aligned with a poor recovery process and prognosis. If nothing has worked so far it is important to go back to the evidence to understand a few main features of how low back pain manifests. Reliance on steroidal or non-steroidal medication in this phase should be avoided because it is masking a mechanical issue in the spine that must be addressed either with PT or surgery depending on the extent of the symptoms. Surgery is rarely more beneficial in the long term than PT. It should only be considered as a last resort to eliminate LBP, specifically if concomitant with severe nerve pain down either or both legs.

During this phase of recovery it is important to perform a regular aerobic exercise program in order to supply oxygenated blood flow to the muscle tissues surrounding the spine. Your spinal discs get their nutrition through osmosis, and the best way to secure a healthy spine is through weight bearing exercise. Squats and walking are both great examples of weight bearing exercises. It is important to consider form and alignment in this phase if you have a history of LBP, as improper form may exacerbate symptoms. Understanding that a consistent, moderate intensity exercise program is paramount to reduction of reoccurrence of symptoms in this phase is crucial and cannot be understated.

What To Expect For The Future

If you suffer from chronic LBP, you are probably thinking to yourself, "Is this ever going to go away?" The answer depends on how you implement the strategies from this book. Eliminating chronic LBP is difficult and requires changes to multiple facets of your life. Implementing even just a few of the aforementioned healthy habits will allow you to decrease your risk for reoccurrence of LBP. Due to its complex and often non-specific nature, LBP treatment does not allow for a one-size-fits-all approach. In fact, quite the opposite is true. A targeted approach to overall wellness is key, including nutritional assessment, weight-loss (if needed), appropriate sleep regimentation and proper exercise prescription.

What about genetics you ask? Sure, genetics do play a role in your risk for DDD and other arthritic/ inflammatory components of LBP over time. That does not mean that you can't do everything in your power to counteract the effect of genes on your daily life and function. Powerful research shows that exercise reduces morbidity and mortality rates associated with chronic LBP. If you can find an exercise regime that works for you stick to it. It may just save your life!

CHAPTER NINE

NECK AND SHOULDER PAIN

Is it Me or Does Everyone Get Neck Pain?

The prevalence of neck pain among the general population in the United States is considered to be upwards of 50% per year. That means that 1 in 2 of us will experience some sort of 'kinked' neck, whiplash or other neck injury this year due to a myriad of factors. There are different types of neck pain, but by far the most common type seen in my clinic is referred to as 'mechanical neck pain' and occurs when the joints get stuck causing difficulty in rotating the neck in one direction or another. Neck pain may also be present with referred pain down your arm, or may be combined with a headache or dizziness. These are common problems I address often. Let's define some common risk factors to see if you are predisposed to neck pain.

Risk factors for chronic neck pain include:

1. Being female
2. Prior history of neck pain

3. Age (> 40 years old)
4. High job demands
5. Being an ex-smoker
6. Low social/ work support
7. Prior history of LBP

If you fall into any of the above categories, chances are you have experienced neck pain. Most people try chiropractic therapy first, with some success. Others turn to their PCP and subsequently to a branch of medicine known as physiatry to get a cortisone shot to quell the pain and symptoms. Often this does not provide long term relief, just as we spoke about with the knee. Cortisone shots will have only ephemeral positive effects if the underlying mechanics of the pain are not addressed. The underlying mechanics include range of motion of the facet joints of the neck, as well as the strength associated with its surrounding musculature and mobility of the joints involved. If you are suffering from neck pain the first step to recovery is a proper physical examination to address your specific neck mechanics.

We have established that most people will get neck pain, so let's talk about why, and what you can do about it.

Can Neck Pain Cause Headaches?

Tension headaches (cervicogenic) are a brand of headache associated with tightness of muscles in the back of the neck. Often this is a result of poor posture or what we refer to in the clinic as *upper crossed syndrome (UCS)*. UCS is often seen in those who sit at a desk for long periods of time. UCS is also common among knitters or weekend warriors that focus too much on working the 'glamour muscles' and neglecting the back of their bodies, while at the gym. Luckily, stretches and some gentle manual therapy will eliminate your headaches if the genesis is tight sub-occipitals. How do you know if the muscles in the back of your neck are tight? Try this test. Bend your neck forward, if your chin cannot reach your chest without a pain or severe stretch of the back of your neck then the sub-occipital muscle group should be addressed.

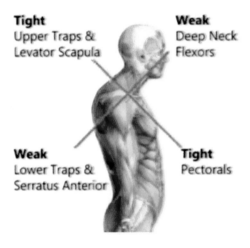

If your posture looks like this, please call a PT!

Is Numbness and Tingling Down My Arms Bad?

Pain referred down your arms is called radicular pain, and can come from a kink in the bones of your neck or tight muscles in that same area. If the pain is constant, or you experience shooting pain or dizziness please contact your PCP immediately. Most likely one of the three major nerves that innervates the muscles and sensory mechanisms in your arm is being compressed by muscle or bone. To put your mind at ease, call your local PT who will easily be able to tell if that is the case for you. I have included several nerve glides in the appendix that you should try if you have radicular pain down your arms. These exercises will keep your nervous system mobile and reduce your risk for aches and pains as you get older.

The Room Is Spinning! What Do I Do?

The first thing to properly distinguish here is this: is the room spinning or are you lightheaded? As medical providers, there is a big difference in the way that we examine and treat both symptoms. Lightheadedness is often associated with low (or sometimes high) blood pressure and may get worse when you stand after sitting for a period of time. This is called orthostatic hypotension, and is more common as you age. Have you ever gotten up quickly, taken a few steps and became lightheaded? If so, then the chances are you have experienced a slight bout of orthostatic hypotension. Dizziness may also occur from something as innocuous as a change in medications or a new prescription for eyeglasses. This is different than dizziness in a spinning form, which is associated with vertigo. The most common type of vertigo we deal with in the PT clinic is Benign Paroxysmal Positional Vertigo or BPPV for short. Nausea or vomiting can also be associated with vertigo and may last for hours or days before resolving.

BPPV is best treated in the outpatient PT setting. You will know you have BPPV if the room is spinning around you. You will get a feeling similar to the one you experience when leaving a boat. The spinning is usually temporary, but may be more severe in certain cases. The spinning sensation typically occurs when rolling over in bed or when sitting up from a lying position. Luckily, it can be successfully treated by a licensed PT with several positional movements and a period thereafter during which you keep your head and neck upright for 24 hours.

Think And You Shall Become

Have you ever been in the position of hiring an employee? If so, would you be looking for a candidate who arrives for the interview with a positive attitude or one who is sullen? One who is articulate or one who mumbles? One with good upright posture, or a person with slouched shoulders? My guess is if you run a successful organization you would want someone with a confident stature to represent you and your ideals. My point is that having proper posture goes beyond preventing injury. Proper posture is tied to many other important markers in life including overall salubrity, success and mental well-being. Your outlook on life is vastly different when your spine is aligned correctly. Let me explain.

There is a theory in psychology called the *self-validation theory*. In a study published in 2009 Brinal et al. discovered that the way you sit determines how you see yourself, positively or negatively. Study participants yielded either a confident (upright) or doubtful (slouched) posture. They wrote down positive attributes about themselves and were then asked to rate themselves on a series of confidence measures. You guessed it. Those with tall confident postures rated themselves as happier and more competent on all tasks.

Take-away: Think and act confident about a goal or task and you will be more likely to accomplish it!

How can you create a healthy posture? The first step is to use a mirror to become aware of your current posture. I suggest taking a picture of yourself from the front and the side. Try not to "pose" for the camera and capture your normal posture as close as you possibly can. You must have an awareness of your current posture before trying to change it! In the appendix of this book, I have added exercises that will help you build a stronger core, spine and posture. To start, try to lift up your chest and become more aware of how you present yourself. I suggest setting a phone reminder to repeat every hour at your workstation entitled "posture!" As soon as I say the word "posture" in the exam room, people immediately sit more erectly. That is your brain's subconscious way of saying, "oh ya, I knew that!" Most of us have the ability to sit up tall, but lose the battle to gravity over time. That is avoidable and correctable. All you need to do is become aware of the problem and do strengthening exercises to fix it!

Link Between Posture and Shoulder Girdle Pain

Shoulder girdle pain is often caused by poor posture. The etiology of many shoulder injuries is poor shoulder blade movement on a kyphotic mid-back (thoracic spine.) Most of us acquire an exaggerated thoracic kyphosis from being sedentary, performing jobs requiring long periods of sitting, or slouching day after day. The hunched (kyphotic) posture reduces the small space in the shoulder where the rotator cuff muscles insert and ultimately increases fraying and tearing in shoulder tissues and tendons. Shoulder symptoms that begin as small tears and slight impingements can become full thickness tears and potential surgical cases. There is strong evidence to suggest that performing a shoulder blade strengthening routine will prevent injuries from occurring. Performing a specific shoulder strengthening routine will also reduce risk for surgery, even if a labral or rotator cuff tear has already been diagnosed.

What are some tips to both improve posture and reduce neck and shoulder pain? Enter our next healthy habit. This habit is one that I've been telling my patients to do for years. You can never perform enough of these!

Healthy Habit Winning Rule #8: Perform 10 'Chin Tucks' at every stop light. This will improve your posture and reduce your shoulder and neck tightness.

The primary exercise that I prescribe for neck and shoulder pain, with a proverbial gun to the head, is a chin tuck. I will include how to properly perform this exercise in the appendix under Neck/ Shoulder exercises. You should know that your upper trapezius muscle group is innervated by a cranial nerve, and tied directly to your limbic system. Your limbic system stabilizes emotion. When you are experiencing higher than normal levels of the stress hormone cortisol, your upper traps will subconsciously begin to contract. This propagates the elevated shoulder and increased muscle tenacity noted in the following upper crossed syndrome picture. The chin tuck strengthens the anterior muscles of the neck which are often overstretched, while at the same time stretching and contracting the upper traps to improve your posture and realign your ear lobes over your shoulder blades.

Here is a fun fact: for every inch your head is placed forward over your body, your body (upper traps primarily) is lifting a lot of extra weight! I have included a visual of this below. The average bowling ball is 16 pounds, imagine having to hold a bowling ball with your neck muscles everywhere you go!

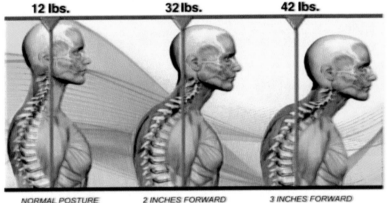

12 lbs.   **32 lbs.**   **42 lbs.**

NORMAL POSTURE   *2 INCHES FORWARD*   *3 INCHES FORWARD*

Tips to Improve Your Neck Pain

The first recommendation I suggest to my patients, after having a thorough examination and evaluation for neck pain, is to index when and where they are experiencing neck pain and to record their symptoms. Often people lose track of the amount of time they spend sitting in front of a screen perpetuating a poor forward head posture. My second tip for reducing neck pain is to recognize your exacerbating variable, i.e sitting in front of a computer screen for 5 hours a day.

Range of motion, specifically a lack of it, is another key contributing variable in the development of chronic neck pain. You lose about 1 degree of neck rotation per year after the age of 26. So if you start with 90 degrees of neck rotation in each direction, by age 86 you have on average only 30 degrees of rotation when turning your head side to side. To put this in perspective, if a patient presents to my PT office lacking 45 degrees of rotation to a particular side, they qualify to be referred for an X-Ray to see if there is a more noxious cause underlying their pain. The theme is to work on your neck rotation while you've still got it! It is easy to perform just a few neck stretches 3-4 times a week. This should ward off stiffness that is associated with age-related changes if you are religious with the habit of stretching.

Stress is the last main contributor to neck pain primarily because of its ties to the limbic system. Stress creates the release of cortisol causing your upper trapezius muscles to contract. This passive contraction leads to suboptimal movement patterns of the spine and shoulder girdle and remains the etiology of much neck discomfort. Mitigation strategies for stress include understanding what is causing the stress in the first place, and then taking action to reduce it. The action you take will depend on what is causing the stress, and may have nothing to do with strengthening muscles or stretching joints. Numerous variables can contribute to your stress levels. You might be in a poor work situation, have a sick loved one, or be experiencing financial difficulties. Action to mitigate the cause of the stress will require intervention more substantial than just stretches and strengthening. A more seasoned physical therapist understands the eccentricities of the body and knows that not all physical problems are solved in a conventional cookie cutter way.

It is important for your medical provider to take a thorough medical history in order to properly diagnose and understand your situation in its entirety. More information is needed, not just simply how your neck moves. With a more thorough understanding, you will have a better grasp of what steps and habits you need to take or change in order to ameliorate your neck pain once and for all.

Conquer Neck Pain Associated with Headaches

How about those who suffer from headaches and migraines? What can a book about healthy habits do for them? Cervicogenic headaches are a common occurrence, and a primary reason for referral to a physical therapist. Headaches that occur in the back of your eyes or to your forehead are what we refer to as "Ram's head" distribution of pain. They often indicate the genesis of the headache is from tight sub-occipital muscles. Often the solution for these headaches and migraines might be as simple as finding the right pillow to sleep on or performing a couple simple stretches to ease the tension in your neck. But how do you know that it isn't something more? Try this simple trick: Turn your head. If you cannot turn your head forty-five degrees to the right or left then it is time to go see your PCP or local physical therapist. Research shows that an X-Ray is required to determine if degenerative changes are in play if you have very poor rotation mobility. Often curing neck pain and headaches is as simple as adjusting your reading posture or limiting the amount of time spent sitting at the computer. Sound simple? Success with healthy habits should be!

Tips for Achy Shoulders

If I had a quarter for every time I was approached for a consult because of painful overhead reaching, I would be retired already! Shoulder impingements, labral and rotator cuff tears are very common. Shoulder pain can happen to anyone, at anytime, but specifically occurs more often in the later stages of life (>50+). In fact, a study reported that 51-54% of people between 60-80 years of age have a rotator cuff tear. The incidence of shoulder pain later in life is greater because your small rotator cuff muscles get less blood flow as the body ages. Less blood flow to the rotator cuff tissue in combination with fatty infiltrate of the muscle tissue and age related sarcopenia is a recipe for disaster. Most people won't take action until they either realize they cannot pick up anything from a top shelf anymore, or their shoulder starts to hurt constantly.

Shoulder pain could be coming from a variety of sources: radiculopathy from the neck and spine, adhesive capsulitis (frozen shoulder), ligament/ tendon tears, impingement, labral tears or possibly a tumor or fracture. It is best to consult with a PT or your PCP if you are experiencing constant pain that is unrelenting and unmitigated by non-steroidal anti inflammatories (NSAIDS) or Tylenol. If you have pain that is intermittent, and low to moderate on the pain scale, I suggest you try some of the exercises in the appendix or refer to my website https://conciergephysicaltherapy.com/shoulder-pain-free-report/ for more detailed information.

In order to improve your shoulder symptoms, understand that like any other muscle, the shoulder needs consistent resistance training to stay healthy. Resistance training for the shoulders is of particular importance because often the directions we move our shoulders performing daily routines are limited by poor posture and bad habits. In order to start with a clean slate to fix shoulder pain, postural correction is key. I will address that next. Since I am providing general information in this book let me preface my remarks by saying that you should be seen by a movement specialist (PT) if your pain has been going on for longer than 2-3 weeks. Go ahead and try a few of these habits for healthy shoulders and download the free report from my website - https://conciergephysicaltherapy.com/shoulder-pain-free-report/. What do you have to lose?

Shoulder Pain and Posture

The link between shoulder pain and posture is inextricable. Very rarely does shoulder pain coincide with perfect posture, and vice versa. There is a strong correlation between poor posture and shoulder pain. To explain, your shoulders work in a 3-D motion, with your shoulder blade as its base of operations. If you have poor posture, chances are your shoulder blades are tipped forward, crowding the rotator cuff interval and space in the shoulder joint that allows you to achieve full ROM overhead. If you are skeptical, try this trick.

> Slouch, and try to reach your arms all the way overhead. Have someone take a picture of you from the side. Next, sit up tall and do the same. Compare the pictures.

This activity will put into perspective the relationship of posture and shoulder ROM. If you have poor posture, chances are you are **losing up to 60% of your available shoulder ROM**. As the old saying goes, "if you don't use it- you lose it!" With all that loss of motion, your scapulae start to reposition and you are left with internally rotated shoulder blades and a minimal amount of space for your rotator cuff muscles to do their job of stabilizing the shoulder joint. See the pictures below for details. You want to be in a posterior tilt, external rotation position. So how do you get there? Use the pictures for reference.

BAD	GOOD
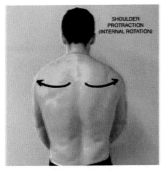	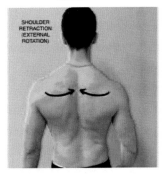
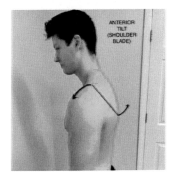	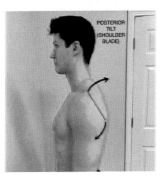

Healthy Habit Winning Rule #9: Do three pulling exercises for every one pushing exercise at the gym, at least 3 days a week.

My Muscles Are Torn, Now What?

Let's say you have been diagnosed with a rotator cuff tear. You can still lift your shoulder away from your body (it isn't fully torn requiring surgery) but it is incredibly painful. What can you do to manage your symptoms, pain and debility, in order to improve the problem? The solution is to begin to exercise the muscles in your back and rotator cuff.

When you work the muscles in the back of your body and your rotator cuff, you will start to improve the dynamic forces in your shoulder. The lower trapezius, rhomboid and infraspinatus muscles in particular play a huge role in symptom relief in non-operative shoulder rehab. Unfortunately, often times these muscles get overshadowed by the glamour muscles that we can see in the mirror and often overtrain: the upper trapezius and pectorals major. Your job is to avoid allowing the pecs and the upper traps to win the strength battle! The strength battle between the front and back of your body is an endless war. If the front of your body wins, it is almost always associated with poor outcomes for your neck and shoulders! Heed my advice and perform three back exercises for every one chest/ pushing exercise, and incorporate this into your weekly *healthy habits* routine. Your neck and shoulders will thank you and me!

CHAPTER TEN

EXERCISE AND STRETCHING SAFETY MANUAL

When was the Last Time You Could Touch Your Toes?

A regular stretching routine can do wonders for an aging body. Not only does stretching reduce your risk for injury but it can also improve your energy and calm your mind. Stretching is a regular part of most physical therapy treatments in my clinic. Almost everyone benefits from the implementation of a daily stretching program which improves blood flow to your muscle tissues and tendons, allowing more oxygen and nutrients to enter. Stretching also helps to improve your posture and reduce your risk for injury by increasing your muscle length.

It is important for your muscles to be able to achieve required range of motion (length) when called upon. Let's take golf for instance. If you spend most of your time sitting at a desk in an office, chances are your hips and low back are tight. A tight core makes it difficult to make a full rotation during a golf swing.

While you may not experience immediate pain from golfing, unless you perform a regular mobility routine, you almost certainly will experience discomfort in the future. It may take months or even years to develop, but the pain will occur. Over time, pain and compensatory strategies will affect your swing path decreasing your ability to score well. Why not fix the problem before it starts with a consistent stretching regime tailored to your overall health and well-being?

How Long Do I Need to Hold a Stretch?

I am often asked questions regarding stretching. For example: Which stretches are the most important to do and in what order? How long should a stretch be held? How many days a week should it be performed? What is the point of warming up before stretching? Prescribing a generalized stretching routine is difficult because everyone has different needs. I will use the average baby boomer and recent retiree as an example.

It is important to complete a self-assessment first to gauge where you stand before we begin. I have a myriad of self-assessment techniques on both my Facebook and Instagram pages if you are interested in more details on understanding your personal flexibility baseline. The purpose of the self-assessment is to identify muscle groups that may be tight which pertain specifically to you. This way you can spend more time stretching those muscles rather than other muscle groups that are already flexible. If you do not feel comfortable with self-assessment, make an appointment with a physical therapist. My staff periodically perform personal Functional Movement Evaluations to provide patients with personal movement tips. I would suggest taking advantage of the opportunity to have a professional assist you.

I have identified no less than **10** stretches that almost everyone would benefit from doing everyday. These stretches target those from the baby boomer generation, but can be performed for good health maintenance cross generationally. Remember, it is always a good idea to consult with a PT or PCP prior to starting a stretching routine or performing any of these exercises.

Healthy Habit Winning Rule #10:
Stretching should be performed 6-7 days a week and all stretches should be held for at least 1 minute.

Prior to a stretching routine I always recommend warming up with gentle aerobic exercise for 8-10 minutes. Performing some light aerobic exercise lubricates the joints and increases your heart rate and vasodilatation (blood-flow.) Better blood-flow to your muscles is crucial to improve the ease in which your muscles will retain their newfound malleability. It is important to note that the way your body retains muscle length is by following up with specific strengthening exercises to reenforce a mind-body connection. The "mind-body" connection is what many call "muscle-memory." This memory is the ability to use neuroplasticity and brain chemistry to improve your ability to move the way you want to. If you have never worked out before, there is a period of nervous system adaptation that has to occur for several weeks prior to your muscles being able to grow in size.

When stretching, your nervous system has to ramp up and be worked to capture your new found muscle length. Adaptation then occurs in order for your brain to understand what your muscles are capable of. To "work" the nervous system we follow stretching with several specific strengthening exercises that we refer to as "neuromuscular re-education." These exercises enhance the mind body connection and improve your motor control which help to make the positive changes to your muscles during stretching, permanent.

Using a baby boomer as an example, let me outline an order of stretches that would be extremely beneficial for overall health and well-being.

1. LTR's
2. Posterior Pelvic Tilts
3. Hamstring Dynamic 90/90 Stretching (B)
4. Prayer Stretch
5. Prone Press Ups
6. T/s Rotation (B)
7. L/s Rotation (B)
8. Cross Arm Stretch
9. Cat Cow Stretch
10. Piriformis stretch (B)

*(B) denotes stretches to be done bilaterally, or on both sides And if you have plenty of time add these:

1. Hip Flexor Kneeling Stretch (B)
2. Calf Stretch (B)
3. Plantar Fascial Mobility (B)
4. Quadriceps stretch (B)

Pictures of all of these stretches are included in the Appendix. Try not to get overwhelmed with the number of stretches that should be performed daily. Instead focus on the ones that you derive the most perceived benefit (stretch) from. Again, if you are looking for a mobility baseline I would suggest having a Functional Movement Screen performed at a PT clinic near you. You can then note your progress every 2 weeks or so. This will add to the momentum of your positive new habit. Try to devote 10 minutes every morning to stretching and keep a diary of how you feel when you are done. Compare your thoughts on day 14 to those of day 1, reflecting on the progress you have made.

Health Benefits of Regular Yoga

Yoga is an age old practice that encompasses movement and mindfulness in a manner that is beneficial for the body at any age. When you channel good thoughts and are able to focus on the present moment, your body is able to reflect on its needs. Surveys from a Harvard University study indicate that those who practice yoga are more satisfied and less critical of their bodies. Those who practice yoga also exude better decision making in the kitchen by choosing healthier ingredients when preparing meals. The benefits of performing a yoga routine at a minimum of twice a week include:

- Better Body Image
- Improved Mindful Eating
- Cardiovascular Benefits: Decreased Blood Pressure, Cholesterol, Blood Sugar
- Overall Fitness and Flexibility
- Weight Control

The more you practice mindfulness within your yoga sessions, you will notice improved mood due to gray matter changes in your brain's Amygdala. The Amygdala is the "stress" center of your brain and shrinks on a fMRI scan with consistent practice of mindfulness and yoga. Correspondingly, gray matter density increases (cortical thickness) in the hippocampus and pre-frontal cortex. With increased grey matter density in these two areas your body benefits from improved:

- Focus and Concentration
- Emotion and Impulse Control
- Self-Awareness and Recognition
- Ability to Evaluate Rewards and Consequences
- Ability to Delay Gratification

If you have time, add a yoga routine for an hour to two a week to your schedule, and reap the benefits of better decision making, improved impulse control and better body image!

Tips for Those Who are New to Exercise

Let's take a moment to touch on some of the parameters to consider before beginning an exercise routine. It is always wise to consult with your physician if you are new to exercise in order to determine if there is anything exercise related that you should be careful of. This is for a variety of reasons. Many of us may have minor hereditary conditions like Marfan's Syndrome, systemic joint hyper-mobility, or more serious conditions like an abdominal aortic aneurism that would limit our ability to exercise in an "all-in" fashion. It is also a good idea to have a lipid profile taken if you are overweight so you can determine the objective effects of your exercise. This will mark a baseline for your progress. When the results of your bloodwork improve, it will be another accomplishment for you to celebrate!

A few things happen to your body when you start working out. The first thing that happens is your nervous system kicks in to adapt to the new movements that you are introducing to your body. This is somewhat similar to learning a new language. Your body needs to process and adapt to the changes that are occurring within it. This is the Neural Adaptation Phase, and occurs when your body is improving the ability of the motor units to deliver electrical impulses to your muscles and ligaments. Neural Adaptation occurs throughout your life when you learn new activities and sets the groundwork for your body to lay down new muscle tissue.

It may take several weeks for your body to adapt to exercise. During this time you will experience no muscle hypertrophy (size) changes! This is normal.

During the next phase, that I deem the Hypertrophy Phase, your body will begin to gain muscle mass. *Muscle mass is key to reducing your risk for many sports related injuries.* The amount and fiber type (fast twitch or slow twitch) of that hypertrophied muscle tissue will depend upon how you workout and stress your body during exercise.

What Happens to My Muscles During Exercise?

During the exercise itself it is important to understand what is happening to your muscles. When you perform any variety of the exercises, similar to those done in a PT clinic or elsewhere, you are actively *breaking down your muscle tissue.* Your body then activates various hormones including testosterone and HgH to quickly rebuild this muscle to match the *stress* with which you challenged it. The key note is: if you are not working into muscular fatigue or stressing your tissue it will not change! When you are done working out and specifically while you are sleeping at night, hormonal levels increase, resulting in the greatest amount of muscular healing. It is imperative to have the proper amount of protein in your diet for muscle generation. Protein is the building block of muscle tissue in the human body. How much protein to consume is always a topic of hot debate. To be safe you should consume at LEAST .8 grams to 1.5 grams of protein per kilogram of body weight depending on how active you are throughout the day.

Response to exercise will vary slightly from male to female. Due to their hormonal landscape, men have more testosterone and HgH making it easier to build and retain muscle mass. Your body's response will also be dependent on how you load it and what variety of exercises you perform.

How Much and How Often?

I'm often asked the question: "Dr. Lordan, how often do I need to exercise in order to experience the benefits of doing so." The first thought that comes to my mind is *as often as possible.* However, it is not that simple!

Specifically, *how* you work out will determine what your body will look like after a period of a few months of consistent exercise. My suggestion is to start with a personal trainer if you are brand new to exercise, and have them develop a routine for you. A trainer will teach you the basics of exercise (safety, muscle groups, etc.) so that you do not injure yourself from the get-go.

They will also devise a plan based on your goals: strength, toning/coordination, weight loss, balance, or a combination of the aforementioned. The training *style* (think sets and reps) will vary based on the goals you are looking to accomplish. In the exercise world, this is what we call a loading effect. In order for your body to change it needs to adapt to a new stress to create that change and improve. Nothing good comes easy. It takes work (stress to the muscles!). If you have experience in the gym and are comfortable getting started on your own, I recommend the following outline of the basics of training styles as a general template.

If your Goal is:

Strength: 3 sets x 12 reps; 75% of your 1 Rep Max; 4-5 times per week

Toning: 4 sets x 20 reps; 30 - 50% of your 1 Rep Max; 5-6 times per week

Active Aging/ Balance: 3 days of 45 minutes brisk aerobic exercise (3-5 / 10 on a scale of exertion); 30 minutes of a balance + exercise routine put together by a PT; 3-4 times per week

Weight Loss: 3 days of aerobic exercise 30-60 min (5+ / 10 on scale of exertion); 3 sets x 15 reps; 60- 75% of your 1 Rep Max 3 days a week

*You can find which weight to use by benchmarking your "1 Repetition Max" here: https://strengthlevel.com/one-rep-max-calculator.

Your Journey To A Healthier You: Healthy Habits Streamlined

Viewing beautiful models and actors portraying characters on the film screen when you turn on your television set may find you saying to yourself, "Why can't I look like that?" The fact is that most of those people have strict routines and diets that enable them to look that way. It is an all encompassing journey of wellness that includes mindfulness for mental health, proper nutrition, exercise, daily movement and a myriad of other variables that some folks have already created into a healthy habit 'streamline.' Now it is your turn.

What is a healthy habit 'streamline?' It is a build-up of inertia that I spoke about earlier. Now that you have the knowledge it is time to put it all together to create a happier, healthier *you*. We spoke about mindfulness, and the power of stacking daily habits in order to maximize will-power reserves and use inertia to our advantage. We talked about the multitude of injuries that try to sabotage our path to wellness, and what to do to fix them. Finally we touched on ways to get the results you are looking for depending on your specific goals and desires. Everyone is on a different path to wellness and all are at different points along their journey. Do not rush it. Enjoy and learn from the new knowledge that you have acquired from this book. I challenge you to implement 2-3 healthy habits, and then find ways to stack and optimize them in your own life.

I would enjoy hearing from you via email about the benefits you have received and the progress you continue to make.

CHAPTER ELEVEN

THE TRUTH BEHIND THE CONCIERGE PT APPROACH

Three Truths of Physical Therapy

At the time I am writing this book, I have practiced physical therapy in a myriad of clinical settings for the better part of 15 years. In those 15 years, I have had the pleasure of working in a variety of settings all across the United States (hospital, in-home, Concierge PT, outpatient orthopedic sports medicine and skilled nursing, to name a few). During the past decade I have worked with a range of ages and conditions from infants with torticollis to nonagenarians who can barely get out of bed. The vast exposure that I have had has given me some enlightenment on three basic truths of physical therapy, and what it takes to achieve a successful outcome for both the patient and provider.

1: Physical Therapy is NOT easy

Showing up to PT is just the beginning of the process. Most do not even get that far. With the ease of seeing a PT without a doctor's script today, there is no excuse not to simply "show up" for a consultation with a PT. I hope after reading this book and learning about direct access to PT services that more will be comfortable making a direct call to their local PT if they have any musculoskeletal issues. That being said, once you enter the door of a PT clinic, the fun starts and the work really begins.

The first step of any PT evaluation is to obtain an answer to your health problem. If it is a muscle ache or pain, I can tell you with 99% certainty that your local PT will not only be able to help, but if they cannot, they will send you to a specialist who can. That is what is wonderful about today's Doctor of Physical Therapy programs around the country. They teach students how to "rule-out" red flags in order to make sure it is safe for the patient to move forward with physical therapy. Ruling out red flags also coincides with recommendations for further imaging or potential Physiatry or Orthopedic involvement. We refer to other professionals when deemed appropriate and vise versa. However, usually (at least at my clinic) it is we who refer to the orthopedics, physiatrists and PCP's because we see people first. That is not the case everywhere, but it happens quite often where we are located.

Now, after you have an answer to your health problem, in the form of a diagnosis and a prognosis, is it time to spring into action. This is the part that we, as PTs, call our "Plan of Care (POC)." The POC is developed on an individual basis and is, in a way, a contract between patient and provider stating that each will do their utmost to achieve the desired results. The follow through with the POC is the most difficult aspect of PT, but ultimately the most rewarding. Successful POC completion requires excellent camaraderie between both patient and therapist. I require all of my PTs to be trained in Emotional Intelligence and stress the importance of rapport. Without it, the chances that a 10-14 week POC will be completed are negligible. That is sometimes how long it takes to get well. In this regard, completion of the PT POC is difficult and requires a high level of communication and commitment from both parties. Throughout the implementation of the POC a combination of some or all of the following will occur: manual therapy, exercise, dry needling, ultrasound, electric stimulation, and hot/cold therapies. All of these interventions and modalities require some level of effort from each participant (patient and PT) and require a high level of trust between patient and provider in order to sustain the most effective outcome. Usually it comes down to asking yourself this question: "Am I willing to continue living my life without being able to _____ ?" Then: "What am I willing to do to *reach my goal /eliminate the pain / sleep at night?*" Do you wonder why I say: "PT is not for the faint of heart?"

2. Physical Therapy is a PRIMARY solution to muscle aches and pains

Years of helping people solve their chronic pain problems such as those who have previously been addicted to medications or who have suffered failed surgeries, has taught me one thing: PT needs to be the first intervention for anyone suffering a musculoskeletal condition. When I say "musculoskeletal" I am referring to common joint aches and pains caused by trauma, chronic overuse or aging, or a myriad of other culprits. I wish I had a nickel for each time I heard the comment, "I went to the PCP and they told me to rest and apply ice, but it just never got better."

Why didn't that person think of PT as a solution? Is it because we do not promote our solutions to common problems like LBP well enough? Is it because the PCP truly does not think PT can help or that they think it is a waste of time? Does the patient think that PT is ONLY a set of exercises, or just the application of some electric stimulation pads with ice placed on top? I still do not understand why a physical therapist is not thought of as "PCP" for LBP or general muscle aches and pains. Hopefully this book will help to shed light on the solutions PTs can provide, as well as save patients time and money by eliminating the visit to the PCP by coming directly to physical therapy.

That being said, it is also important that any PT treating patients, some of whom are walk-in patients, be versed and well educated in medical red flags and symptom patterns. I urge patients to research their providers to make sure that they are well respected in their community. Doctors of Physical Therapy are in the unique position of providing tailor made solutions to societies' most common muscle and bone ailments. If only more people knew!

3. Physical Therapy will test your resolve to determine how committed you are to getting better

"No Pain, No Gain." Have you ever heard this mantra before? Those who have been through one or several bouts of PT know and understand this phrase well. We have established that PT will get results for those who have musculoskeletal ailments. What we have not touched on is the mental fortitude required for patients to get the results they desire. The first thing that most people want when they come to PT is to be able to perform an activity that they are no longer able to do, such as: walking, climbing stairs, or golfing. The reason they cannot perform the activities they love is because they are hampered by pain, decreased range of motion (ROM), and concomitant muscle weakness. A PT will work with you to address the impairments, pain, ROM and strength, in order for you to be able to return to doing what you love. However, as I've said multiple times throughout this book, it is not that simple! A tremendous amount of dedication is required from both the practitioner and patient in order to achieve the goals of the PT treatment plan. Your desire to "get better" through PT will always be in competition with the perceived easy road (surgery, pills, or shots) even though these interventions oftentimes just mask the symptoms and do not address the root cause of pain. What is scary is that, potentially, the ROOT cause of musculoskeletal pain is nowhere near the site of impairment!

Follow me here. Those who suffer from chronic LBP typically present to PT in a sinusoidal fashion over the years with bouts of "good" times as well as "bad" times. The difference between the good and the bad days usually consists of a few tiny habits that mount up and are not noticed until the pain becomes unbearable. Initially it may be a slight pain in the back that eventually becomes a radiating pain down the leg. Maybe it is an extra 10 pound weight gain that shifts the posture forward causing premature degenerative changes in the low back due to increased facet joint load and increased articulation. Minor habit changes can have large effects on pain cycles.

Would you believe me if I told you that calf tightness causes back pain? Probably not. Truthfully, the funny thing is that calf and hamstring tightness actually both play a large role in the incidence and occurrence of both low back and knee pain! Try this simple drill as a test:

1. Do a Body Weight Squat
2. Do a Body Weight Squat with your heels up on a 2 inch step

Does one version feel easier than the other? Is it much easier to squat lower and with better balance if your heels are propped up? The step assists you in reducing tension in the back of your legs. You can also reduce tension in the back of your legs by stretching! The better you are able to move the less pain you will have.

Why the Success

"What makes Concierge PT different?"

In this context, I am often asked about my Outpatient Sports Medicine practice in Massachusetts. What makes my practice different than others is that we follow a central assessment method based on the bodies intricacies that is easily replicated from person to person. This central method has a focus on patient-centric goals and outcomes and relies on the Doctor of PT to identify not only the source of the problem (the easy part) but to get to the root cause of the issue (the hard part).

'Regional Interdependence' is a term that I like to use to define how we uniquely define our assessments. Initially coined by Suieki et al. in 2013, 'Regional Interdependence' refers to the confluence of factors that affect how a person moves and feels. At Concierge PT we recognize that eliciting a positive outcome is not as simple as treating one joint or body part at a time. For instance, even though you may be experiencing pain in your spine, the root of the pain may not be the spine at all!

After identifying the anatomical pain site (example: LBP), the next step is to do a thorough movement assessment to figure out what other impairments of muscles and joints exist in the body. This involves identifying the tissue that is creating the noxious/painful response in the body. As we have established, the impairment that is causing the pain is usually away from the site where symptoms are present.

The next assessment layer entails achieving a high level of camaraderie with the patient to understand the underpinnings of their specific psychological situation as well as potential medical yellow flags that may be contributing to their current status. A yellow flag may be poor nutrition, high stress levels, or even an inability to afford treatment at the recommended allotment. The list goes on. In order to find the source of the pain, we need to understand our patients on a level deeper than simply asking: "Where does it hurt, and how long has it been going on?"

The success at Concierge PT is due primarily to our PTs ability to identify and treat the true origin of the pain. Often the true origin of pain (key restriction) is 2-3 joints away from where symptoms reside. This is due to the interconnectedness of the musculoskeletal system as a whole.

By approaching our patients with a 'birds-eye view' perspective, we are able to eliminate pain at a systemic level. We have a strong referral network in place to make sure patients get the attention they deserve in areas like nutrition and mental health. This leads to exceptional results and often less time in active treatment leaving you more time to devote to doing the things you love!

The Concierge PT Regional Interdependence Model

Let's take a moment and discuss the intricacies of the Concierge PT effect. The premise is this:

> Fixing the root cause of aches and pains is the key to eliminating pain without risky surgery or reliance on medication and is best attainable through the Concierge PT Regional Interdependence Model.

How is the ankle connected to the shoulder and neck? How is the spine connected to the knee and to the arch of your foot? How likely is it that a headache is caused by tight hamstrings? The only examination model clinically proven to identify such connections exists... within Concierge PT Regional Interdependence Model (CPTRIM). Through implementation of the CPTRIM we are able to greatly reduce the risk for painful surgeries and push patients to become medication free in as little as a few weeks.

Rewind to the year 1977. The "concept" of Regional Interdependence (RI) was born when Dr. Richard Erhard discovered something astonishing. Dr. Erhard discovered that all regions of the body appeared to be linked; but that is not all. In order for his patients to recover faster and at a higher level of function, he had to take into consideration how the other bodily systems (brain, sensory, emotions) are linked to muscles and bones. Consequently, interventions that focus on a single structure or body part often result in a poor outcome. What was inferred before is now peer reviewed and scientific fact. A total body assessment is key to ascertaining the "big picture" and fixing the body at its root impairment. This is the secret behind the CPTRIM, and why it works so well.

The Real Problem in Medicine Today

Using the contemporary modern medical approach, "treat when ill," there is a shift away from the real problem: addressing the risk factors before they turn into something pernicious. The *real problem* plaguing our healthcare system is that risky surgeries, overmedication, massages, pain patches and occasional trips to the chiropractor or PCP will not address the root cause of a patient's symptoms the majority of the time.

Sure it may feel nice to have your back cracked, but there is a reason why you have to go back every week to get results. There is a reason why a "pill" is never a panacea and will not give you lasting results. It only masks your symptoms and makes you feel better for the short term. A pill does not address the underlying motor neuron/ psychological or sympathetic response to pain, nor does it identify and create symmetry in the body in order for pain patterns to finally be resolved for good. Only a model focused on the big picture will identify all factors associated with creating a salubrious, natural outcome for a patient.

In fact, if you are trying pills, medication, or surgery but still not getting the results you are looking for, it is not your fault. It is because all other healthcare providers are focused on the location of the symptoms, not on the root cause of the problem.

It is because the root cause of the problem creating your symptoms has yet to be diagnosed... until now. The breakthrough technique at Concierge PT is totally different. Our regional interdependence model is a brand new way of assessing the human body. The CPTRIM focuses on fixing the cause, not treating the symptoms, to finally get the solutions you have been waiting for. Solutions that will keep you active and healthy well into old age.

Who is to Blame?

Have you ever been told, "Just rest, ice, and it will surely go away on its own?" If you have, you are not alone. You are a victim of the "cookie cutter" chain PT practice experience. Sure, rest and ice may work for some, but that advice is not tailored to your specific needs, nor to your specific desires or goals. If you truly want to live a healthy and active lifestyle well into your 80's, 90's, and beyond, then it is time to distance yourself from the terrible advice offered at "chain clinics." Those clinics see you more as a number than as a human being.

No more settling for sabotaging advice like "rest, ice, and it will go away." No more "just do these 3 exercises and you'll be fine; no need to see me again. It is time to take a stand for your health and future! It is time to address the ROOT cause of your pain.

Why Should I Make a Change Now?

I want you to mark on your calendar the first day of the month following your purchase of this book. This "New You" day is the day that is going to thrust your expectations to the next level. It is the day designated for you to start your new personal "New You Resolution" wellness journey. Do not wait! We know how often "resolutions" are actually followed through to fruition! But, once you decide to go all in on improving your health and try our regional interdependence method, you will not look back. I urge you to make a choice NOW. Make a decision today to start your new wellness journey. As I have mentioned previously, every wellness journey should have solid habits, and goals. If you never get assessed using the thorough Regional Interdependence Model we employ at Concierge PT, how will you achieve them?

Why Should I Trust You?

You may already "know me" having seen me on television, in the newspapers, or on the internet as a contributing columnist for health magazines and newspapers nationwide. Or perhaps you have watched podcasts and interviews where I'm frequently invited to share my opinions on current trends in the field of PT. However, I didn't start there!

I started my PT Career back in 2006, when I joined the American Physical Therapy Association as a student PT. From there I moved through Northeastern University's Accelerated Doctoral Program in Boston, MA, acquiring Board Certification in Orthopedics a year later. I have spent the better part of the last decade perfecting a treatment approach different than conventional techniques utilized in the past. Currently, I am fortunate to be able to share the Concierge "Secret Success" formula with the world. That is my passion and life's calling.

I learned in short order that there was a noticeable standardization of treatments that patients were receiving from one clinic to another. The treatment model I have created will help anybody, not by providing "cookie cutter" exercises aimed at treating symptoms which many PT clinics offer, but by using the RIM model. In fact, my approach has already helped thousands of people, just like you, to improve their quality of life and resume the activities they cherish.

I invite you to check our website https://conciergephysical-therapy.com/reviews/ for testimonials. It is an honor and a privilege to spend my life helping people. If you know someone who is sick of treating their daily aches and pains with medication and rest, send them this book! It may change their life.

Benefits of the Concierge PT Care Model

Your health and future is at stake. The average person seeks healthcare for a mere 100 minutes a year. Is that enough time to devote to your health? What happens during the other 525,500 minutes of the year?

Facts:

1. Less than 45% of Americans get the recommended amount of physical activity in a day
2. 70% of Americans are considered to be at an unhealthy weight
3. 70% of Americans do not get enough sleep
4. 75% of Americans have experienced anxiety, depression, insomnia or fatigue due to life stressors in the past year

The facts above define the recipe for a health disaster. As recently as 2014, the US Army made sweeping changes by switching to a largely holistic model of healthcare. Holistic health practice involves addressing the person as a whole, not simply treating one issue or body part at a time. The US Army is now taking a preventative "holistic" approach to health and wellness. What can you learn from them? It is better to address the root cause of disease by looking at the whole picture before it becomes a much larger problem.

In order for you to begin to understand how the Concierge PT Method works and how it ties into holistic care, you need to understand how the body works. I will give you a hint... its not in isolation using only certain muscle groups. Your body is a complex organism that requires communication between cells and body parts. Simply put, you need the combination of a healthy mind, body and soul in order to live the best version of life you are capable of.

Therefore the only solution is to have a thorough 'holistic' examination of the weaknesses (muscles, nutrition, stress etc.) that are sabotaging your health and wellness. Those that are decreasing your likelihood of living healthily into your 80's, 90's and beyond. I am talking about quality aging and enjoying a life that does not require the assistance of a walker, wheelchair or worse.

The Concierge PT Model is a system that focuses on your specific weaknesses in order to successfully steer you and your loved ones into a worry-free future. A future devoid of the numerous physical ailments that haunt many of your less enlightened contemporaries. The best part is that a consultation with a Doctor of PT is only a phone call away.

Healthy Habit Winning Rule #10:

Schedule a thorough movement assessment, and establish a mobility baseline. A physical therapist at Concierge PT will accomplish this and more.

The key is to address the symptoms of disease before they become a larger problem. This is best achieved through a holistic healthcare approach and a thorough yearly physical evaluation. At your evaluation, the PT will identify tight muscle tissues and abnormalities that will lead to a myriad of issues down the line, if left untreated. What if you could prevent being one of the 4 in 5 people who suffer from back pain throughout their lives? I recommend having a thorough movement assessment. Isn't that worth an hour of your time?

Avoid the "Cookie-Cutter Chain PT" Practices

We have been over how you probably have been told: "Just rest and ice. Your pain will go away in a few days." Or my personal favorite: "It will go away on its own. Just stay out of the gym and don't do any exercises for a week or two." Have you ever been to PT for a lower body injury? Perhaps you looked around the clinic and saw everybody doing the same exact exercises? This is the classic "Cookie-cutter chain PT" clinic.

This is a typical scenario combining bad medical advice with care given by a busy local provider who lacked the time to do a thorough medical examination on each patient. One who did not develop individual plans of care. This bad advice is not even the biggest problem facing the field of PT today!

Usually it is one of three different scenarios that occur at busy chain PT clinics. Hopefully you or someone you know has never had any of the following experiences at physical therapy.

Scenario #1: You show up day one and receive an evaluation from a PT who maybe does a little massage. Then you are led through some exercises. You are not instructed about the nature of your issues, nor are you told exactly what to expect from therapy or the timeframe it will take to fix your problem. You may get some ice on your knee (where you said it hurt) and are sent on your way. No follow-up visits are scheduled. You just receive some printed exercises and a business card with a number to call if things get worse.

Scenario #2: You show up day one, have a thorough evaluation from a PT, get some massage on the affected area and are educated on your treatment plan. You then proceed to show up for several more sessions where a PT Aide or assistant will walk you through 3-5 exercises that are already on your home exercise sheet. Then they perform ultrasound or electric stimulation on your affected body part before sending you on your way. Maybe the PT checks in, but does not perform hands-on therapy on you again because he is too busy and is seeing too many patients. This lasts perhaps 4 or 5 sessions. Then you decide that you can do the exercises on your own at home and don't need the help of a "PT" anymore. You think: "What were they doing to *help* anyway?"

Scenario #3: After receiving a quick evaluation from a stressed out, busy PT who explains that next session will be different when he will have more time to spend with you one on one. Unfortunately, at the next session there is a mix up at the front desk or with scheduling and you end up with a PT Assistant who just brings you through 30 minutes of exercises and puts some ice on your problem area at the end of the session. The next few visits go much the same. You see a PT or PT assistant for about 30 minutes at a time, but never the one who did the initial evaluation on you to begin with. You are stuck not knowing whether you are making progress. You feel like you could just do the exercises they are showing you at home, so you decide to do that instead.

This is how business is done at 99.9% of PT clinics (even some of the ones I have worked at in the past!) Now let me show you what you can expect from a visit at my outpatient PT clinic: Concierge Physical Therapy.

The Concierge Difference

After having a wonderful conversation with a member of the front desk staff, you will begin to feel like part of the Concierge PT Family. The receptionists take pride in *understanding you and your medical problem, without having met you face to face!* The receptionist will take fastidious notes and put them in your patient chart for your Doctor of Physical Therapy to review prior to your initial visit.

Upon arrival, you will be greeted with a smile and offered a cup or coffee, tea or water in a warm, friendly, clean environment to make you feel *at ease.* Your Doctor of Physical Therapy will then greet you, introduce themself, and bring you to the examination room for a private comprehensive evaluation. You will be given plenty of time to explain what is occurring that brings you to PT. Your Doctor will explain exactly what to expect from your rehab and discuss a time frame to fix your problem.

Together, you and the doctor will develop a plan of care to address your issues. Your PT will set the expectation for how long it will take to improve your pain, and then address the root cause of your problem in order to restore function and reduce the risk of further reoccurrence of the same issue(s).

You will receive a folder upon leaving with a list of your future appointments as well as a sheet explaining the exercises you are to perform over the coming weeks (if applicable.) It is our aim that you will leave feeling better than you did when you entered the clinic because your PT will have done some hands-on manual techniques to reduce your pain at your very first session. These techniques are often combined with electric stimulation and or other advanced manual techniques that we perform concomitantly to control and reduce pain.

Over the coming weeks you will see the same Doctor of PT who performed your evaluation, or you will see a DPT who specializes in your problem area who will work in conjunction with your evaluating PT. During each visit, you will have hands-on treatment focusing on healing your muscles, tendons and joints to improve your symptoms and decrease your pain. Soon you will notice that your pain will start to lessen, just as your PT said it would at the beginning of the process.

Typically, about 4-6 weeks into the process you will start to have days where you experience no pain at all! At this point, your PT may change the treatment plan a little bit depending on their findings during a specialized re-evaluation to begin to focus on the root cause of the pain that brought you to PT in the first place. The goal being to assure that the pain does not come back in the near future from one wrong turn or twist.

At discharge you will be given a party favor reminding you of the accomplishments you achieved by successfully completing your PT plan of care. We've given out coffee mugs, t-shirts, *yetis*, to name a few, to serve as a memento to say, "Congratulations, you did it!" Since you have developed a fabulous rapport with your PT and the staff at Concierge, you might receive a card from the staff wishing you well on your life's journey. You can't put your finger on it, but the experience was outstanding and well worth the effort.

This is the "Concierge" difference. Please do not settle for anything less.

Who is the Right PT for You

At Concierge PT we understand that everybody is in a different stage of their journey. With that said, in the physical therapy world there are a number of sub-specialties that the general public is not typically aware of. I will briefly mention a few of the sub-specialties that we offer at Concierge and what you should look into.

The first rule of thumb is to look for board certification. Any free-standing outpatient clinic you choose should have a manager or owner who is board certified in Orthopedics, Sports, or Pediatrics- depending on what specialty of care you are looking for. The following are 9 board certifications in PT:

-Geriatric, Pediatric, Orthopedic, Sports, Neurology, Cardio-Pulmonary, Clinical Electrophysiology, Oncology, and Women's Health

I am not saying this is a must for the clinic that you choose, but if you have a specific issue that may be more complicated, a clinic that has specialists will be more likely, in my opinion, to help you to achieve a successful solution to your problem. If you have a Women's Health issue, then you will obviously go to a women's health specialist (we currently serve Women's Health needs at Concierge PT). If you have had a complicated orthopedic surgery or have suffered with lingering back pain for years, you should probably seek out an orthopedic expert. It makes sense to choose an orthopedic doctor over a general practitioner.

Many PTs graduate now with Doctorate degrees and will be very capable of treating many disorders. However, there is a significant difference in continuing education among therapists. Make sure to peruse a clinic's website to become acquainted with your PT prior to seeing them. Come to your first session prepared with questions about your condition and your chosen PT's experience treating it.

CHAPTER TWELVE

CONCLUSION

Summary of the Healthy Habit Winning Rules

Following the 11 rules for a healthier lifestyle will be no small feat. These tools are meant to be a guide for you to begin your health journey. The moral of the story is: make a few small changes to improve your quality of life and live a happier tomorrow. Here is a summary of the rules again.

11 Winning Rules

You must use will-power first to make a positive decision affecting your health. Then inertia will help make this positive change *permanent*.

1. Use will-power to make a positive decision that will affect your daily life.
2. Get out of bed ONE hour earlier each morning and spend the time doing something you ENJOY.

3. Say your Prayers and/or Meditate for 10 minutes before bed each night. Watch the quality of your sleep improve immensely.
4. Log the time you spend on activities for (3) straight days. Then carefully analyze what you can eliminate to make more time in your day.
5. Try something new that you have been hesitant to do before. Your brain will reward you for it.
6. Start small and follow the 2x2 rule. Start with 2 positive habits and implement a small change over the course of 2 months.
7. Take a 30 minute walk or bike ride, or workout vigorously twice a week for 45 minutes.
8. Perform 10 'Chin Tucks' at every stop light. This will improve your posture and reduce your shoulder and neck tightness
9. Do 3 pulling exercises for every 1 pushing exercise, at least 3 days a week.
10. Stretching should be done 6-7 days a week and all stretches should be held for at least 1 minute.
11. Schedule a thorough movement assessment, and establish a mobility baseline. A therapist at Concierge PT will accomplish this and more.

How Implementing the 11 Rules Will Change Your Life

According to a study at Duke University, habits account for about **40 percent** of our daily behaviors. If you can implement even small changes, perhaps just a 1% daily growth, your life will be positively affected. We talked about many strategies to improve your will-power and to stack good habits for the best overall effects. By implementing just 1 of these rules, your life will change for the better over the long haul.

For instance, let's say you choose to implement only the 4th winning rule, which states:

> **Log the time you spend on any activities for (3) straight days. Then carefully analyze what you can eliminate to make more time in your day.**

Let's say you spend 4 hours looking at your cell phone screen each day. Instead, spend that time on your wake up routine, exercising, creating a less hectic work schedule, and being present with your loved ones. Imagine what adding **12 hours** to those three days might do for you. You would most likely improve your relationship with your family and loved ones because you now have time to do so! That is only one of the benefits of reflecting on your daily and weekly routine. There is always time to be found. Your job is to match it up with your goals and the activities you value.

Personally, I value family time and my health. When I look at my 3 day routine, which I do about 2x a year, I look for more time to reinvest in those two categories. I might add a family game night on Friday evenings, or spend 1 hour on a Sunday afternoon to prep meals for the week. It does not matter what you choose. All of our values differ, so choose something meaningful to you. What does matter is that you take a conscious look at how you spend your time. Then change it for the better.

Consistency is Key

Repetition builds habits. It is that simple. When you find a habit pattern that works for you, stick to it! Keep it simple at first, then evolve by slowly beginning to stack your habits while making other positive changes. The best part is you will begin to get a dopamine rush from feeling better mentally and physiologically. This will contribute to cementing your good habits. The toughest part is sticking to your new routine. We are all human, and it is easy to slip up by abandoning a routine. Vacation is the perfect example. We think: *"It's only a week. What's the worst that can happen?*

To be truthful, the chances that you resume making the healthy shake you were making in the morning, after the 14 hour fast, prior to vacation is slim. The good habit is harder to implement upon returning home! We have all been there. We tend to trudge back into the workweek after a fun packed vacation and forget all of the positive changes we made prior to going. Do not let this happen to you! A good way to avoid this is to set a calendar or phone reminder for the day you get back saying: "Don't forget; make a shake this morning with avocado, almond butter, protein, honey and cinnamon. Don't drink it until 10:30am!" The more specific the better. And if you have *Instacart* or *Amazon* deliver groceries to you the night before, you will be all set for the morning. Make it easy to choose healthy habits and you will make better choices more often than not.

Benefits of Having a Health Coach

Working with a "Health Coach" is one of the best decisions you can make. A good health coach will guide you with a preventative holistic approach to care that will help you meet your specific health goals. For example, while a physical therapist will help determine the root cause of your knee pain by looking at your whole body and how you move, a good health coach develops a plan and creates goals for you based on sleep, nutrition, stress and a myriad of other factors.

The first thing a health coach will help you do is identify your specific health goals based on what you want out of life. There are many aspects to a healthy lifestyle, so determining specifically what is most valuable to your success is crucial to a salubrious outcome. Most folks do not realize what they want out of life until they reflect on it with some guidance. A health coach will create initial action steps for you to take to fulfill your long term health goals. The most common goals being: symptom and disease management, weight loss, improved mental health, and creating an overall healthy lifestyle that is sustainable and rewarding.

A health coach will also fill the knowledge gaps related to nutrition, sleep, psychology and my personal favorite: debunking myths! A common myth in the health realm is:" fat is bad." Fat is not intrinsically bad for you and the macronutrient is an important part of your diet. There are different types of fat that absorb and breakdown for energy utilization at different rates to complement other micronutrients and macronutrients. Unfortunately many fad diets give fat a bad connotation. Mainstream media makes it even worse! Fat may be the one thing missing from your diet that will help you feel better, think better and move better! However you will not know this until you consult a health coach with a nutrition background.

It seems most people are confused about what, how, and when to eat in order to fulfill their nutritional needs. We are surrounded by false advertising claims such as "heart healthy" and "low carb" products that are portrayed as being the healthier option. The fact is they are making us fat and sick. Regulations about what goes into our food and onto the labels of our food are so vague that it is very difficult to know whether the food we are choosing is good or bad. We benefit from certain ratios of micronutrients and macronutrients. With some of the popular ways of eating, we are missing out on important aspects of a healthy and well- balanced diet. Your health coach will help you to wade through the information options presented to figure out what, how, and when to eat to support a healthy body, reduce inflammation, balance your hormones, and so much more.

Self-discovery is another tactic employed by your health coach to help enhance your life's journey and reach your personal goals. Valerie Feghali, a licensed Health Coach and Doctor of PT say "Balance and consistency are key to a healthy lifestyle, and your health coach will help you achieve this with accountability and mentorship."

Can PT Help You?

The most common question that I get as a Doctor of Physical therapy is: "Does physical therapy actually work"? What a loaded question this is! I say this because it assumes that the PT clinic you go to employs the same core values and ideals that we, at Concierge, do. The core values of care and ideals at Concierge PT stem from offering a holistic approach to your symptoms and problem. We address the root cause of your movement dysfunction and fix the problem by addressing the cause, not just your symptoms. Typically the "Does PT help"? question is asked by someone wrought with skepticism from battling a long fight against a chronic musculoskeletal disease, such as low back pain. This same person has probably had PT in the past with minimal success, most likely, because the focus was placed on getting the back moving without addressing any of the adjacent tissue restrictions preventing the back from moving in the first place. Probably, this person has resorted to Aleve, Tylenol, Cortisone Shots and perhaps narcotic medication or even surgery in an attempt to get rid of their nagging back pain. My advice, try PT. After all, what do you have to lose?

What Do You Need to Do to Get Started?

If you live in Massachusetts, I advise you to pick up the phone and call Concierge PT. A Doctor of PT versed in our specialized holistic assessment method will be able to give you a thorough movement examination and get you feeling better right away with hands on massage and exercises.

The best part? You can see a PT without a script from your doctor. This is true in MA but can vary state by state. You do not need to be in pain, nor do you need to have an "injury" to see a PT.

A good PT will guide you through a series of steps to activate muscles and joints that are tight, preventing you from becoming injured. If you do not live in Massachusetts, this book is an excellent guide to getting started on the road to a healthier you. I wish you luck wherever your health journey takes you.

I love to hear from my readers. Please feel free to reach out with any health related questions or concerns you may have. I am currently quite busy in patient care, but I will get back to you as soon as I am able!

I end this book with a notable quote that moves me each day:

"Yesterday is history, tomorrow is a mystery, today is a gift. That's why they call it the present." -Tamara Levitt

APPENDIX

(Images Available At conciergephysicaltherapy.com under "Book" Tab)

Shoulder Exercises:
B ER w band
Sidling ER w DB
Serratus Pushup
YTI

Neck Exercises:
Chin Tucks standing
Scalene stretch
Upper Trap Stretch

Low Back Exercises:
Piriformis stretch (figure 4)
Prone Press ups
Prayer Position
Bird Dogs
Cat/ Camel

Knee Exercises:

Clam Drop Outs w Band
Bridges DL / SL
SLR w VMO bias
Lateral leg raises
Squats with Band

Foot/ Ankle Exercises:

Short foot towel grab
Marble pick up
Calf stretch
Great toe extension
Eccentric calf raises
Plantar fascia release

Nerve Glides for Numbness and Tingling:

Median Nerve
Ulnar Nerve
Radial Nerve
Sciatic Nerve

Made in the USA
Middletown, DE
03 May 2023

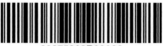

29875908R00082